Link to Life

Spinal Cord Injury

Link to Life

Spinal Cord Injury

Contributing editor: Lydia Thomas
Series editor: Kevin Mulhern

B⬛XTREE

CENTRAL

Dedication:
This book is dedicated to the memory of Jillian Duguid

First published in Great Britain in 1994 by Boxtree Limited

The 'Link' Programmes are produced for Central Independent Television by Coffers Bare Productions Limited

1 2 3 4 5 6 7 8 9 10

A CIP catalogue entry for this book is available from the British Library

ISBN 1 85283 905 8

Cover designed by Design 23
Text designed and typeset by Wilcom Services
Printed and bound in the UK by Cox and Wyman for
Boxtree Limited
Broadwall House
21 Broadwall
London SE1 9PL

Contents

Preface vii

Introduction xi

Ian Martin 1

Ellryn Ashdown 15

Mike Marten 25

Judith Jesky 45

Tim Marshall 65

Stephen Bradshaw 95

Preface

Back in 1982 I was asked to leave my job at the BBC and work for commercial television's 'Link' Programme. At that time 'Link' had been on the air since 1976 and my immediate reaction was to wonder how much longer it would have to run: unlike the BBC, commercial television was ruthless in ending series long before viewers had tired of them. My guess was that 'Link' had perhaps another three years before it was brought to a close and so I left the BBC and became its producer.

Today 'Link' is still on the air and has become a permanent feature of the ITV Network. 'Coronation Street' is the only networked series on ITV which has been around longer. 'Link' was then, and still is today, unique amongst television programmes. It is the only regular weekly television programme, anywhere in the world, aimed specifically at a disabled audience. It is also the only programme exclusively researched, written, presented, directed and produced by disabled people themselves.

'Link's longevity and its success has much to do with the philosophy behind the programme, and how it originally came into existence. Back in the mid-1970s Richard Creasey, 'Link's first producer, was asked to put together a short series of documentaries about disabled people. After researching for several months he told the network controller that disabled people did not want another series about them, they wanted a series for them. Creasey had detected in the disability community a deep desire to stop turning out the usual run-of-the-mill programme about what it was like to be disabled. Then, as now, most television programmes portrayed disabled people as either hopeless victims or superheroes.

Audiences were asked either to feel sorry for disabled people or else admire them.

'Link' decided to portray disabled people as they really are – as a part of our society, not apart from it. One in every four families has a disabled member and disabled people are husbands, wives, partners, parents and children. They are in reality like any other individual, but they happen to have a physical or mental impairment. The programme does not ignore the fact that Britain's six and a half million disabled people face enormous problems: problems of discrimination, of poverty and a lack of job opportunities. Where 'Link' differs in its approach is where it puts the responsibility for those problems. The mere fact that one is either born, or acquires a disability shouldn't mean that you are excluded from places of work or entertainment. The fact that disabled people are often excluded is a reflection on the way our society responds to disability.

Some years ago the Department of Social Security initiated a survey to estimate the different categories of disabled people in Britain; it wanted to discover what proportion of the six and a half million could be described as seriously disabled. One of the most significant tests they applied was whether a disabled person could use public transport. At that time a close friend from Berkeley, California was studying in London. Under the criteria of using public transport she was seen as seriously disabled because she could not use buses or trains, at least she couldn't use them in Britain. At home in California public transport was accessible and she had no problems as a wheelchair-user getting around Berkeley or the greater San Francisco area. Her physical impairment remained the same whether she was in London or California, but the environment changed and it was her environment which effectively disabled her.

'Link' has always attempted to explain to both disabled people and to the general viewing public that you cannot view disabled people as a separate part of the community. When town planners, architects and politicians begin to mould our environment they have to remember that disabled people can either be included or excluded. To ensure that disabled people are not excluded, the voice of disabled people has to be heard.

Link to Life is the first series of books to which the 'Link' programme has lent its name and reputation, despite many offers over the years. We have done this because *Link to Life* offers disabled people an opportunity to say how and why they live their lives, and to say this in their own words, unedited by the posse of professionals which often surrounds disabled people.

It is fitting that the first of these books deals with spinal cord injury as this was the topic on which the very early editions of 'Link' concentrated. It is also fitting that the book's contributing editor, Lydia Thomas, is a former presenter of the programme. All the contributors to this book were once non-disabled, people who lived their lives unaware of the physical and attitudinal barriers which disabled people encounter. The discovery that because you suddenly have to use a wheelchair you can no longer visit your friends or go to the cinema has made people who are spinal cord injured great campaigners for the rights of disabled people. Anger and frustration can prove very constructive forces when you are trying to get laws changed and building codes altered, and the Spinal Injuries Association has always been in the vanguard of such campaigns.

The disabled reader will find in these pages comradeship and warmth as well as help and advice, but above all they will hear the clear voice of experience.

But what will the non-disabled reader gain? My hope is that readers of this book will discover that we, disabled people, inhabit the same world as they do. However we often have to use our ingenuity, skill and cunning to live our lives to the full. I hope that the reader will also discover that living one's life as a disabled person is a fascinating and intriguing experience, but not a tragedy and certainly not something to fear.

Kevin Mulhern
August 1994

Introduction

There is often, after a traumatic experience, a hunger and need to know more about others who have been through a similar pattern of events and that's what this book explores: life following spinal cord injury as seen through the eyes of six very different people.

Their injuries occurred over a timespan of three decades so the recollections give a very clear overview of change and development in the perception and treatment of people with spinal injury. The timespan almost mirrors my own experience: I was injured in 1965, aged eight, when I fell trying to complete a somersault during the warm-up for my regular Saturday morning ballet class. The fall meant that I became paralysed from the waist down and I spent about nine months in hospital, initially in the Queen Elizabeth Hospital in Birmingham. My consultant there was a lovely man called Mr Brodie-Hughes. I remember clearly two things about him – that he smiled a lot and was kind. Not qualities shared by all in the caring professions I have since found!

Hospital care and treatment come under scrutiny in this book because unlike some other disabilities the initial stay in hospital after injury is a fairly lengthy one involving a strenuous rehabilitation period. There are good and bad accounts here although Ellryn Ashdown, at 15 the youngest contributor to this book, writes 'I don't like doctors. They're not very good at giving you all the information. If you have a problem they try and put it in such a nice way that you don't understand what they're saying or they put it very bluntly and you still don't understand what they're saying.'

A case of damned if you do, damned if you don't, but as doctors at all levels of the medical profession have a crucial and valuable input during the first months of paralysis and beyond, it's worth emphasizing here that awkward communication skills and lack of empathy with people's real lives are cited on more than one occasion in these accounts. This is a failure of care that can and must be improved within all of our spinal units.

Equally architects, developers and planners, housing associations and others need to take account more visibly and actively that disabled people still want to and have a right to live and work in appropriate buildings, as Ian Martin pointedly writes: 'Although I've achieved a lot by my own efforts I'm still often stymied by practical problems such as access. That manifests itself more as a problem because I get angry with it. I know there are rules that architects have to follow and fire regulations but those rules make life harder for us all and stop us doing things. For instance, if developers build 52 houses they'll proudly say they've made two of those wheelchair accessible. What they haven't worked out is that those wheelchair people can't go around to see their neighbours because they can't get into their houses.'

Inequality within housing, transport and access to public places for employment, leisure, education and the general acts of everyday life lead most of the contributors to argue forcefully for all-encompassing anti-discrimination legislation. At the time of writing it is still quite legal in the UK to discriminate against people purely on the grounds of disability and it is now, more than ever, vital that the full force of the law is used to prevent this, to enable all disabled people to have equal choices and opportunities on a par with non-disabled people. To offer less is indefensible.

Of course, there is much here in this book that's about the ordinary side of life – time after a spinal injury is not made up purely of encounters with medics and bureaucracy, far from it. There is much, much more in our lives than that. I think that perhaps Ian Martin's philosophy rather neatly sums things up when he writes, 'My accident was more of a comma than a full stop. My life didn't change, it just took on a different colour.' If there is a message here to others who have or are close to someone with a spinal injury then possibly that's it, although in reality most of us don't see ourselves as messengers, we simply get on and live, with our disability forming part of what we are.

This books gives much to celebrate and reflect upon. It's honest and forthright, offering a fresh insight into the many facets of our different lives with a warmth and clarity that I hope all who read it will enjoy.

Lydia Thomas
Summer 1994

Ian Martin

Ian Martin was born in 1960. He works as a graphic designer, and lives in Buckinghamshire with his girlfriend. He was spinally inured in 1986 as a result of a ski-ing accident in Austria.

I suppose right from the start in Austria I was expecting to get better, and I think feeling that way was quite useful. When I say 'better' I mean I was expecting to be able to walk again, but when I got to Stoke Mandeville hospital in the UK, the consultants were actually quite keen to get me off that track immediately. They were quite abrupt in their prognosis and said, 'Hello, good afternoon, Mr Martin, did you have a good trip from Austria? By the way you're not going to walk ever again!' They were quite adamant that that was my prognosis, but I could still see that my body was working really hard to cope with what I'd done to it, and I was still gunning for it. I felt that I couldn't let it down just because a consultant told me that I'd never walk again. I'm not sure if there was a very definite cut-off line, but my determination was quite easily channelled into rehabilitation. So, in hindsight, I feel that it was quite a useful thing to have that amount of enthusiasm, or that determination, and I really quite enjoyed my time at Stoke. The rehabilitation was actually quite challenging.

I can't really remember much about the ski-ing holiday. A group of friends had organized it; I'd been ski-ing with them before, but interestingly, I didn't actually want to go on this trip for some reason. It was becoming more and more awkward actually to fit it in with some work I had on, but they were keen for somebody to make up the group, so I went.

On the day the accident happened I'd just won a slalom race. It was at a ski school, and we were doing an exercise, trying to get down the slopes with as few turns as possible. I didn't turn enough obviously, and just fell over and slid off the piste into a tree, but I remember standing at the top of the slope beforehand, thinking, 'I really don't want to ski any more'. It was very strange, a sort of premonition really, and I thought that I would go down really slowly – that was until I saw somebody else do the exercise well, and thought I might as well carry on with it.

I remember I was conscious. I actually think I really knew what I had done as soon as the accident happened. I didn't really understand spine injuries, but I feel I knew what my prognosis was, and things weren't very good. I remember specifically looking at my feet and they weren't where I expected them to be. I suppose they felt as if they were in the same position as they were before my back broke. It was quite strange. After that, I can just remember that I was watching the ski instructor, watching his training really: he brought a helicopter landing pad out of his knapsack, a little flare and little arrows that he put on the snow. I was just passing time watching that, with people putting coats under my head and stuff, then we had a quick flight to Schladming Hospital. They gave me a tetanus injection and a large bill, and that was it, and then put me back on the helicopter and said, 'I think you'd better go to Salzburg'. I spent ten days in Salzburg and I got on well with the staff. I could speak a little German which the nurses worked out, and they wouldn't speak any English so communication was quite hard. Some of them had learned English at school, and they brought a German/English dictionary in for me to use, so I made quite good friends with them really. The insurance company brought my Mum out there, which was probably a bit boring for her as she was sitting in the hotel most of the time. Then, after ten days, at the end of the ski season, they flew me home. They got a charter flight out to get me home, like a Medevac (there were no direct flights home from Salzburg), and the insurance company obviously thought this was an ideal opportunity to get their name mentioned. I was the local hero in the next issue of the local paper, with reporters bugging my parents trying to get information out of them. I don't know why ski-ing into a tree made me a hero. The headline just said, 'Local hero still smiling after breaking his back with little hope of ever walking again.'

My first weekend at Stoke Mandeville was actually Easter. I got there the Thursday before Easter and I remember my first few days in hospital being excruciatingly quiet. Everybody else went home. I was quite conscious of other people a lot worse off than myself, people who couldn't move their arms and had to have everything done for them, so that made me feel lucky, even though my break is a complete one.

I was in Stoke for five months and I actually enjoyed it, there was quite a good sense of black humour. It made me think of the Guinea Pig Club, at the McIndoe Burns Centre at East Grinstead. It was built during the Second World War. They revolutionized the treatment of burn injuries for pilots and they made the double amputee the treasurer because he couldn't run away with the funds! It was that same sense of humour that I found at Stoke Mandeville. There were a lot of young people whizzing round in these really smart wheelchairs, and things were looking fairly good really.

In Stoke, I listened to Tina Turner a lot, and resumed Spike Milligan's war memoirs. I seemed to have quite a few visitors: actually, I think I held the record for having the most people at one time, about fourteen! The staff were great there, though, very lax on regulations: I had friends with me until midnight on my birthday and things like that, and they were quite happy about it.

Rehabilitation was quite challenging. I found it quite hard work, and I enjoyed that, but I don't think I rehabilitated as well as I might have. I had a lot of opportunities to try archery and some other sports which I found quite fun, but I wasted a lot of the time messing around with another guy who shared my sense of humour. It was a bit of a party really. We were out every night and on late passes, I actually had a visitors' book which people used to write in if they came to see me because I was out so much.

I came out of hospital in September 1986. I went to my parents which was I think a mistake, probably more for them than for myself. I'd actually signed the deeds for a house just before I went ski-ing which happened to be in Aylesbury, about a mile away from Stoke Mandeville, so it was quite a coincidence really. I signed the deeds before I went away, and I actually exchanged contracts while in hospital. My solicitor brought all the information to St Francis ward in Stoke Mandeville for me to complete. He had kindly gone to the building society and said that Mr Martin had hurt his back and would it be all right if he got all the papers for me as I needed a bit of work doing on the house. In the meantime I stayed with my parents for a few weeks until I sorted all those things out. There was very little work left to do. My brother and friends came round and knocked a wall out, widened a door into the bathroom and put a ramp up the front of the house. It was a semi-detached house, so I used to climb up the stairs to bed each night, and just lived downstairs during the day. The bathroom was downstairs. I couldn't climb stairs very quickly, but I could get up there. To start with I used to walk up on callipers, but I slowly stopped wearing them. I remember doing my washing, putting it in a rucksack on my back and calliper-walking upstairs to put it in the airing cupboard. I was at a stage where I wanted to do everything myself, and didn't need any help, but I've definitely slipped out of that. Things that are hard to do I usually get somebody else to do them.

Luckily, I was able to continue with my work as a graphic designer, even in hospital. Friends and colleagues would bring the work in to me. I was freelance at the time of my accident, and I had desk space with a company in Tring, but the office was up some stairs. There were murmurings that they could pay half the cost of getting a chairlift put in, but I wasn't happy using one, and they would have had to put up a lot of money even to pay half. I think it was about £12,000 for the whole thing. I couldn't justify asking them to do that because I didn't know if I wanted to stay there. About a year later, in 1988, I decided to set up a company working with two friends, work colleagues, and I've since sold my share of that.

My accident was more of a comma than a full stop. My life didn't change, it just took on a different colour. I just had to think about things differently, and choose to do different things. I remember lying in bed thinking of all the things that I couldn't do. My physio went to visit her sister in Zimbabwe, and she came back with all these pictures. She went down the Zambezi in a canoe for four days' camping on the river banks, and I was slightly envious that I couldn't do that. And yet I have managed, slowly, to do most of the things I was originally upset about not being able to do. I've been down the Zambezi in a canoe, which may very well have been the highlight of my life. It was quite a stunning experience.

People might disagree with this, but I like to think of myself as relaxed about life. I think the whole world should tolerate each other a lot better and, if nothing else, you should be able to enjoy yourself. I remember once, before my accident, seeing a television programme about a girl with

Stills disease, a very severe form of arthritis. She was so stiff that her mother had to get her out of bed and dress her. She said something that put a lump in the back of my throat, and she was only seven years old. She said, 'What I'd really wish for is to be able to jump out of bed like they do in the adverts,' and there was me at the time being a complete slob, staying in bed as long as possible. That stuck with me. All that girl wanted was something very simple; we owe it to people like her to make the best of what we've got and enjoy it.

I don't think the accident has altered my approach to life that much. I do have to be better at planning things than I used to be, though. I remember one time, before the accident, when I was on my way to Greece on the train. I just looked out of the window and saw a nice mountain and thought I'd walk up it. So I jumped out of the train and did it. I don't have the freedom to do that now. I need to plan and take a car and find out whether you can get up this mountain another way. You can't be as impromptu as you'd like. The older you get, the more you plan things anyway, so I'm not sure if I'd be in the same position if I hadn't had my injury.

I see myself as the same as anyone else, and I think all my close friends look upon me as just another friend. I just have to do things differently, and there are no more negative and positive sides to me than there are to anyone else. Everybody has their down days, though, everybody has things they don't like doing or they're not very good at doing. Everybody has a disability of some sort, whether it's slight short sight or continually dropping things. I've always thought that I'm larger than my spinal injury, and what has affected me more, socially and economically, is lack of self-confidence, although I think I am maybe a bit more self-confident than I was before. No consultant offered me five months in a unit to try and cure that, and it may not be life-threatening, but to me it's more frustrating than my spinal injury.

I haven't always been quite so relaxed about my injury. I've had to find new ways of dealing with other people. When you meet people for the first time, they're not sure how to place you or how to respond to you, so you can quite easily take the lead in the relationship that might be forming. So, in that respect, I think you have a slight jump on people. I remember when I first came out of hospital I used to get upset if I couldn't get upstairs and up steps at the building society, for instance. I had to learn to communicate better with people, especially those close to me, because they might have to go into the building society and ask for what I wanted. I had to be more successful in getting that message across. I also used to get very upset at people staring, especially children in Sainsbury's, but now I try to address it in a different way and try to get a smile out of them. You can take the lead, and make people understand a lot about you, just by facial language. If a child is looking at me now, I usually try and get them to say hello or smile or wave at me, and it's a lot nicer than getting upset.

I know I'm far more relaxed now than I used to be. I'm not sure if this would have happened anyway - with or without the accident. Anyway, I'm pleased it has happened. Like I'm pleased with my garden, and with the house I live in.

I think my worst moments were when I was first in bed. I thought I could help make myself better, and I was actually asking for books to read about spinal injury and the spinal cord so that I could understand it. The only thing that the staff at the hospital would give me was a little book, which I nicknamed How To Be a Good Little Cripple. The worst image in it was this guy sitting in a wheelchair with a cat on his lap looking out of a window on a rainy day . . . . That was an appalling book, and it really pushed me. It was something to strive away from, so I suppose it had its role. Although it didn't make me very happy at the time, I've always wanted to do everything I could to be as far away from that image as possible.

I have managed to achieve a fair amount since my injury. Though I don't do it any more, I suppose my greatest achievement has been learning to calliper-walk, on sticks. To walk again, in whatever way I could, was so important. I think the medical term is first vertical ambulation, which is a lot closer to the truth than 'walking'. It's very hard work, but in the prime of my calliper walking I've walked across Henley High Street in the middle of the night by myself, and not at the zebra crossing either because it was too far to get to. I've walked the whole length of Cairns Airport after I refused to go in one of their wheelchairs because they took my own wheelchair away from me. I suppose setting up the company was quite an achievement. Business is something that I found hard to do, so achieving it was the goal. Once I've achieved something I tend to lose interest in it, so I suppose the achievement is the most enjoyable part of it. Basically trying to sell myself is quite an achievement for me, it's not something I find particularly easy. I'm not sure how this has been affected by the chair, because people react in mixed ways to you in your chair, businesswise: they either think you can't actually be that good at what you're doing, or totally the opposite, and you win their confidence completely. If you're in a wheelchair, and you're actually brave enough to be selling yourself in this position, then you're quite capable of doing a very good job.

I've learnt to ski again which was a big goal for me. I was quite keen to do that, and this year I was actually teaching other spinally injured people to ski. I really enjoyed that, it was great to give something back to the people who'd helped me, so to speak. When I first came out of hospital after my injury, everything was a challenge, so I just had to do it for my own well-being. I suppose that was being sort of manly.

I have, ironically, been called a bit of an old woman on skis, but that was during my second week at ski-ing after my accident - five years after it happened. I do now think, though, that it's not ski-ing that is dangerous, it's the ski-ers. So I've learnt from my mistakes and I ski a lot more carefully than I used to. And it takes a lot of planning. It's very long-winded in terms of getting kitted up and getting on and off the cable cars. There was a guy there who didn't think that disabled people should ski, so he made life as hard as possible for us which we didn't really need as it was quite hard enough anyway. In terms of learning ski-ing it was very easy, the skills are very similar to standing up ski-ing, the difference is that you sit. The position's similar to sitting in a chair. I was quite frightened at first, but I think anyone is if they're learning to ski so I refused to be beaten. But when you point your head down the full way and take your brakes off - it's called shush in the ski-ing fraternity - it's quite a long run, and I was really ecstatic at the end of that. It was one of the best experiences of my life: it was great to do it again, and to be back up on the mountain.

Although I've achieved a lot by my own efforts, I'm still often stymied by practical problems such as access. That manifests itself more as a problem because I get angry with it. I know there are rules that architects have to follow, and fire regulations, but these rules make life harder for us all and stop us doing things. It's things like thresholds on houses, and toilet doors that open into small rooms. For instance, if developers build fifty-two houses, they'll proudly say that they've made two of those wheelchair-accessible. What they haven't worked out is that those wheelchair people can't go round to see their neighbours because they can't get into their houses. If they go out for a meal, they can't use the toilets. The saddest thing is when Prince Charles addressed the Architects' Association and he said, 'It would be good if all architects had spent a few weeks in a wheelchair'. When the Press asked the chairman of the association if he'd do it, he said, 'I might have ten minutes to do that', which wouldn't quite get the point across. It's sad when somebody so important has that sort of outlook.

Sometimes practical problems are turned into outright discrimination by the attitudes of officialdom. I came back from ski-ing in 1992, and I was in Baker Street at seven o'clock in the evening, making my way home from Gatwick Airport by public transport. A friend had been with me until Baker Street, but she left to get her train at Euston. A member of staff came up to me, and said, 'You're not allowed to travel by yourself', so I'm not sure how they expected me to get home. They weren't going to let me get on the train and that made me quite cross: if it's a public service, am I not a member of the public? But they didn't care at all how I got home, and I thought that was quite appalling. Then another passenger piped up and said, 'Actually I'm travelling with him', and I got on and he got off at the next station! In 1988 I went to Hong Kong and I caught the train from Hong Kong and that was 9,000 miles or whatever. Home at Amersham Station the station-master told me that I should have let them know twenty-four hours in advance that I was coming, and had a big go at me. That amused me, but I love taking public transport and I very often use the train to London.

I've had a few physical problems, too. I've always enjoyed good health and I've always expected it from my body, but I do try to give it something back – I try to keep fit, although I'm not that fit at the minute. I try to eat well, so I expect a return for all the care and attention that I give myself. I've very rarely been ill and I don't intend to be ill in the future. Another little negative side which upsets me is insurance companies and, in some cases, GPs not actually understanding what your needs are. If you ring up for car insurance and they ask you if you are disabled, then they just whack 200 percent on top, or they don't even bother insuring you. The amount of miles I've driven since I've been disabled without any problems … again it's lack of understanding.

I do as much physical activity as I possibly can. I've dived since my accident, on the Barrier Reef, in the period when I was trying to prove myself. I've climbed mountains. We went with Back-Up (a sports charity) to Skiddaw in the Lake District, and climbed up that which was quite good. I also had a go at tandem skydiving. Somebody else did all the diving, I was just strapped to him. He rolled out of the plane and I went with him, slung underneath. He jumped from 12,000 feet and landed in a sandpit with a couple of squaddies there to catch us, so it was no problem at all. The biggest problem was getting a GP to give me a medical note to say that I had no heart complaints.

One thing I wish I could do is take a degree or something like that. I don't think I would have the concentration, which I am sad about, but that has nothing to do with my being in a wheelchair.

The thing with Linda, my girlfriend, and all my friends, is that they just accept me as being nobody different. As I was saying before, the wheelchair is not a part of me, it's just a means to get around. I do ask Linda to fetch things for me because it's a little hard, for instance, if we are in the garden and I want something from the house: it's a lot easier for her to get it than me. Nevertheless I think that's bad and I'm being lazy in that respect. It takes quite a lot of concentration for me to stop doing that.

I met Linda soon after my injury. She was a nurse at Stoke Mandeville, but that's not how I met her. It was during my rehabilitation. We always used to go out in the evening, or round to people for tea. The nurses had parties and things, and we used to go down to them. It was a very sociable time and place to be, and I met her pretty much after I'd left the hospital.

My parents took my injury quite well but I don't think I reacted to them very well. They were a lot more hurt than I understood, and recently I've been helping out at relatives' days at Stoke Mandeville when the relatives of injured people come in and ex-patients talk to them. That brought it home to me how tough it might have been for my parents and friends. It's very easy to be self-centred when you're in that situation and to be quite selfish. For instance, I used to get upset with things that frustrated me, and I didn't appreciate that they would upset my parents as well. My Mum thought it was great when I first got out of bed. The first thing she said was, 'Great, I can push you around in a wheelchair', which was the last thing on earth that I wanted. I didn't see it from her point of view, I didn't see that she was wanting to care for me and help me, and I was just being obstructive. As for my friends, most of them just accepted my injury. My best friend at the time of the accident, who was ski-ing with me, I've seen very little of, and he's actually said that he hasn't coped well with it. But I've made some very good friends since then too. Sometimes, my more longstanding friends do things like arrange to meet me in a restaurant, then I get there and find that it's upstairs, and they haven't thought about it: that's not them being thoughtless, it's them treating me as completely normal, which is quite a nice compliment.

Moving house was a real trial. Apart from lack of interest on my part, it was very hard going to see new houses because people obviously get the house set up for themselves: with wardrobes or cupboards by the front door, and maybe some steps that you could build a ramp on. Actually viewing the house might be difficult too. People would fuss to help me in, I generally felt quite awkward, and I also couldn't see everything I wanted to see. It's quite a hard thing for wheelchair users to do. However, I'm quite happy with the end result. Housework I'm not too keen on, though. It's one of the things I'm really bad at. I could excel at it, but I'm very lazy and quite unfair about it really. Linda does a lot more than I do, which is very chauvinist and old-fashioned. I don't think it's anything to do with my injury at all, it's just a bad attitude. The only thing I actually won't ever attempt to do is ironing. I think it's the most wasteful use of human time ever, that's why I've got a crumpled shirt on.

At work, the biggest problem is often lack of space. A lot of studios are very cluttered and very small, and they also sometimes tend to be in attics or somewhere not very accessible. I think the hardest thing about work not specific to graphic design itself, is access into buildings.

I've been very upset about the running down of the NHS. I've been treated very well and very efficiently by the NHS, and I think the people who work within it are usually very well spirited. As soon as you get outside the spinal units, though, there's a lot of misunderstanding even from medical people. Every GP I've had has been very open-minded to my situation, but some of their partners are not quite the same. In general though, the attitude of doctors is pretty good, and I've been fairly happy with it. I don't think they're the best communicators around, and it's quite hard for me to communicate with them. I think you tend to get on best with the people who are allowed to have more time with you, not the consultants, who have got to see everyone and have got very little time for individuals.

Nurses are a different matter again. I think they tend to understand the situation and the problems a lot better than the consultant. The consultant understands how everything works and how the cogs go round and things but from the social and personal point of view, I think the nurses, physiotherapists and ward orderlies are a lot better.

I've never gone in for any alternative or fringe treatments. A lot of people have been to the Dikoul Centre in Moscow, but I like to think that my life, the way I've behaved, the sport I've done, and the things that I do, have actually given me as good an opportunity as if I'd gone to that centre, or at least done that sort of thing. I've just tried to do as much as I possibly can, as close to anything that I would have done before, like building a rose arbour and digging the garden - I think that's as good a rehabilitation as lifting weights!

The idea of surgery to try and reconnect the spinal cord is great. My only fear is that there are going to be a lot of disappointed people. Will there be enough beds to give people operations if they find a cure? If they do draw up a list to get people in, who goes first? If you've been sitting down for eight years, ten years or twenty years, is it physically possible to stand up again? And who will pay for rehabilitation? Is there the money to do that, or is it private care? If it's private care is that not unfair? I strongly feel that it's a shame that these things – and research – aren't paid for centrally, but there's also a limit to what you can buy out of central funds.

I used to play basketball, and now I have been playing tennis. I even had a win at the London Classic two years ago. That's quite a well-known wheelchair tennis tournament which is run annually in Bishop's Park, Fulham. I'm not sure how far I want to push tennis, but I think basketball was quite good because you mixed with a team. I remember driving up the M6 going to a match, and thinking 'this is great'. You feel really relaxed because everybody's the same and there's not a problem. I don't especially advocate joining disabled clubs or anything like that, I think integration is very important, but at that time, quite soon after my injury, I just felt very secure amongst those people. I thought why shouldn't I get on with things, everyone else was.

I went through a stage of doing tricky holidays: I drove up the east coast of Australia and then on to Hong Kong and caught the train back stopping in China and Russia; I've also been to Zimbabwe, but I think I'm mellowing a little, and maybe beaches aren't so bad after all. There's something to be said for lazy holidays. I can't really knock either sort. I'd still like to do a bit more travelling maybe. I'd love to see Nepal and South America. I don't mind the challenge, that's all part of how I've tried to rehab, so that I can do as much as I can. I suppose in the back of my mind I feel as if it was my fault that I'm in this position, so I owe it to myself to have a positive outlook and try to achieve as much as possible despite it. I love travelling, for instance. I think it's the improvization that I enjoy most. There's a bit of that in my job, and I actually like working out and solving problems. How to get on a train or, canoeing down the Zambezi, where on earth do you go to the toilet, those kind of things are quite challenging. Being a wheelchair user in the middle of Africa was much easier than you might think. There was a guide with us who fancied himself as Crocodile Dundee – he opened beer bottles with his bare hands and things like that! He just loved having somebody to look after, so he carried me out of the boat in front of all the girls, and thought that was great. And when you're sitting in a boat for most of the day, there's no sense of disability, you're an equal, but when you're out on the bank in the evening it's a bit hard. Again I think it's the way you look at it that counts: just sitting on the bank watching all these hippos wallowing in that great river, with millions of gallons passing through every minute, makes you stop and wonder what the point of rushing around is anyway.

Some people can be very unhelpful, even when they think they're helping. Let me give you an example. You're getting out of the car and somebody asks if they can help. Despite you saying no, they still try and help you. I think it's a matter of putting them at ease, so they can actually understand you better. It's a communication skill that I need to learn to improve.

I think I'm becoming a more competent manager of my time, but it's hard to say if that's because of my spinal injury. As I was saying earlier, I don't think my life stopped and re-started again under completely new colours. I just think it sort of pinged off at a slight tangent from where it was going before. I think, all in all, I've coped quite well emotionally, with my injury. There are other things that can be more problematic than spinal injury, and if you look around you, everybody's got problems.

I haven't claimed much help from the government in terms of benefits and so on. I have only claimed for mobility allowance, which was sorted out for me in hospital.

I'm not sure if changes in the law to help disabled people would do much good. I don't like the word 'discrimination', but the law about toilet facilities in pubs and restaurants, for instance, does put disabled people at a disadvantage. My understanding in the UK is that restaurants by law have to provide toilets for able-bodied people and if you sell drinks you have to provide toilets, but there is no obligation to provide toilets for disabled people. I think that is a little off colour really.

I think fighting discrimination is the wrong way to go about it. Last summer I winced at a bunch of wheelchair people who made a road block in Central London. I was just thinking about all those hundreds or thousands of people caught in this huge traffic jam caused by disabled people wanting more rights: what were they thinking about us? I think that's a very negative way of behaving. I think the best way is just by being yourself really, and if people want to accept you then they will. A really good way of making people understand you or to come to terms with you, is if you're ski-ing or up a mountain, doing something that they find hard. People in high streets are afraid to acknowledge you or make eye contact with you, but if you're a disabled ski-er or up a mountain in a wheelchair, they'll come right over and talk to you as bold as brass. That's quite interesting, and maybe that's the key. A lot of what I do is about integration: wheelchair basketball is not an integrated sport, but tennis you can quite easily play with a standing, able-bodied player.

The single most important piece of advice I'd give to someone who was newly disabled would be, don't cloud the issues by worrying about things. Just concentrate on your abilities, not your disabilities. I've known people with no limb movement at all and they've achieved great things. Look at Stephen Hawking who's lost movement and speech – but he's become a good communicator.

Self-pity is so negative and self-destructive. You might also wake up one day and wonder where all your friends have gone. The most important part of my rehabilitation was support from my friends and my family, and I think it would be very hard without them. They've accepted me and helped me in a positive, not an overbearing way.

I would certainly like to have children but, like any aspect of life after spinal injury, it's a lot harder and it needs planning. The physical process for collecting semen involves anal stimulation of the prostate gland with some machine that I obviously never see because I'm looking in the opposite direction. Some people might find this process hard to take, in that there's always someone else in the room. It's painless, but it's definitely not the most intimate way of 'making love'. The semen can then be used to inseminate your partner. I suppose it does take away the romantic, intimate side of having children. I'm sure it's harder for Linda in that respect and that upsets me sometimes. It hasn't created problems in my relationship with her. Maybe I'm being blind and not seeing if there are problems, but I don't think so.

If I did have children, I'd see them as an extension of myself and my family. Maybe that's rather a selfish outlook, but with all the effort that we've put into living and all the pressure for us to survive, there must be a reason for it. The only way to perpetuate ourselves is through having children. I think the nicer side of having children is watching them grow up. I find it fascinating watching them, my niece and Linda's nieces and nephews.

At Stoke Mandeville we had lectures about all different aspects of spinal injury, and I voiced my surprise that one of the long-term effects of my spinal injury was a drop in my sperm count. One way forward might be to take sperm from people immediately after the injury, and store it for use later on. I actually asked the lecturer why sperm wasn't collected soon after the injury, and the answer was that it might be very upsetting to some people. I don't think it would be quite as upsetting as not having any children, and I think she was stating a medical point of view. They take plenty of blood from you and stuff like that. It might be upsetting at the time, but it would be a lot less grief than it is now, trying to sort the problem out. It would also be a lot cheaper for the NHS in the long run.

Ellryn Ashdown

Born in 1979, Ellryn attends New Hall School in Essex. She sustained a spinal injury when only eight months old as a result of a road accident. She lives in North London with her parents.

I became disabled when I was eight months old. I was involved in a car crash. As I was so young when it happened, I can't remember what it was like not to be disabled. I can remember my first day at primary school, though. There was a very big classroom, and I came halfway through a term. Everybody seemed to know each other and it was a very big room, lots of chairs. The only thing I can remember is the teacher saying 'Go and position yourself over there', but because of all the tables and desks and things, I just couldn't get through, so that was embarrassing. The first teacher I had was actually quite unsympathetic and all she said was, 'This is Ellryn, she's in a wheelchair and she's coming into our class'.

I was very unapproachable to the boys and girls in my class because of the wheelchair, and I think it took quite some time before I got really involved within the class. Of course some people made fun of me, you always get that. Some of them would run around the playground holding on to my handlebars and I hated it. I know they made fun of me a bit, and there was name-calling.

When I was about eight, a lot of my friends left and it was incredibly different. Out of all the boys and girls in our class there were only four girls and only one of them I liked. The boys were all right although they did keep their distance from the rest of the class, but the girls were quite nasty and kept saying, 'Oh don't talk to her, she's in a wheelchair, she's different, you don't want to be her friend'. The one friend I did have was rather weak-minded, and was easily influenced by other children, which made life rather difficult.

I could participate in most of the lessons – even games. The school was very easy going and you did games if you wanted to. I just remember that we'd play rounders or something and people would run for me; and if they didn't want to then the teacher would run for me. It was very much, well, play football, but if you don't want to, then sit and watch. Often there would be quite a big group of us just sitting and watching.

At eleven I went to secondary school. My parents had quite a difficult time getting me into secondary school: it took about three years to actually get permission for me to go to school in Camden, but I didn't start school late, because my parents started sorting it out early, after their previous experience with primary schools. The people at the secondary school were very much nicer, and it was such a different environment. My disability didn't make much of a difference to them because they'd grown up and were older and, I suppose, more mature in outlook. There was one girl in the sixth form who was very small and walked on crutches, but she left half a year after I came. Some people had friends who were disabled and there was one girl who had a mother in a wheelchair. They weren't particularly sympathetic, but they just didn't think about the difference.

Now that I'm fifteen I'm thinking a bit about the future. I would like to go on to university, though I don't know what I would like to study, or what I'd like to do afterwards. I just like the idea of going to university.

I don't really count myself as being in a wheelchair or disabled. I just take my life from there, and if there's something I can't do, well, I try to do it anyway. But obviously there is an end to things you can do, like I can't really see myself climbing mountains and things although I do try to do most things. I don't go around saying 'Oh no, I'm in a wheelchair, and life's so tragic'. I've never done that, but there are times when you don't feel so happy about the situation. Once I can remember I got very depressed. It lasted for about a week and my friends realized this and tried to help. It was OK. I haven't had that problem since, but just for about a week I was very, very depressed. I felt that life was unfair. My friends tried to cheer me up and everything, and the feeling eventually wore off.

I think I'm a bit more down to earth than I would be if I wasn't disabled, although I sometimes do have mad ideas. Because of my wheelchair, I think I'm more practical, although I'm still quite mad. I think things through more than I would have done. I have to think ahead because I'm self-conscious about my wheelchair, I suppose. If somebody said, let's jump off a roof on a piece of elastic, go bungy jumping, I'd probably say yes. But what about my wheelchair, where would it be – at the bottom? – and that sort of thing.

I suppose I do have to rely on people a lot, which can cause problems with friendships and create barriers. For instance, I'm not often invited to other people's homes because the parents of the child worry about how they are going to manage my wheelchair. Can they get me into the home? Will the wheelchair fit in the car? And all sorts of things like that. As I've come along, though, I've found that people aren't thinking about that as much any more, maybe because they know me better, or they just seem to not mind that I'm in a wheelchair and try and adapt to it anyway. On the positive side, I get in to places half price, for example!

I enjoy doing lots of different things but I particularly love canoeing – kayaking or anything – but I hate boats, and that's a bit of a catch-22 situation! When we go to France we often go canoeing as a family, so it's often me and my sister together in a canoe and I really enjoy that, just the feeling of gliding on water.

I haven't passed any tests for canoeing, or anything like that, I just do it because it's fun. Once I was part of a Camden Council team which took part in a disabled games. I did the track events and swimming. Overall we weren't placed – a second and third, but no firsts – but it was still very good fun. I swim at school too, but because I go to a school for able-bodied people, if we're having matches or anything, very often it's other people that are swimming. I love swimming. It's so different, because if you're in a wheelchair you're sitting the whole time. To get into the pool I just come out of my chair and belly-flop. If you're swimming, you're sort of moving about without having to use your arms – well, you do have to use your arms but you're a bit more free. My sisters don't particularly like me swimming, because I sort of swim underwater.

I had to do work experience with the school as part of our GCSE coursework and we had to find places to do it. About six months previous to that I'd been interviewed for a radio programme and I asked the producer of that if I could do work experience in six months' time. He gave me a list of names and I wrote to all these people and then they put me on to other people. After a lot of letter writing I managed to get a place and I joined the Radio World Service training department, sitting in most of the time on a course which was training journalists. I sort of followed them in what they did. I did so much, because the journalists there were not proper journalists, but were training to be journalists: they were taught how to write in different ways, how to write specifically for radio. Then they had to write a piece and record and edit it and everything, which to me was totally new. I found I was quite hopeless at it but never mind, I still tried and I made programmes, and I wrote despatches and I did interviews, I did everything. I even made a short programme, on who will be the next James Bond, in which I interviewed George Powell, producer of the World Service Film Programme. I did a vox-pop and used a Sony tape recorder and microphone, and I spoke all about who will be the next James Bond, and who people want to be the next James Bond.

I would like to go on radio but I'm very shy and self-conscious about speaking to strangers and meeting new people, so I'm not sure if that would be the best work, although once I do meet people I'm OK. You've got to be pretty good at English and I'm totally hopeless at that, English is not my strong point.

I've been participating in the Duke of Edinburgh Award Scheme which my school runs. I've been doing it with the rest of my year, and it's basically walking and camping. At first I didn't really think I'd be allowed to do it, partly because I wouldn't be able to walk the fifteen miles, but it's been adapted so I've been pushed part of the way and I've wheeled myself part of the way. There are seven of us in the group which is more than the normal amount because of special modifications, and we've been allowed to have seven packs carried. We are going to be walking fifteen miles to Sandon which is a village near our school, and then six months later we are going to be walking on Dartmoor. We will be doing twenty miles over two or three days. The teacher has already done the route. The bits where I can't do it, if there's another way round we'll be taking that, or I'll be driven that little bit by car.

I'm really looking forward to it. I love camping and things like that – eating, picking your own food and sleeping outside – so I think it will be good fun. I've never actually been away with my year before so it should be great. I've been camping before; my aunt takes my sisters and I and a couple of our friends every year for about five days. We camp in Devon where she lives on a campsite, and we have to cook our own food and camp. I'm a very bad cook, so not many people will actually let me cook.

I'm also rather a disorganized person but I'm very particular about my tent, it has to be very tidy, no bugs, no grass.

My Mum just takes my disability in her stride. She and my Dad just treat me the same as my sisters, so there's no difference between me and them.

My sisters are very helpful, they are concerned and worried at the same time. You know, 'Are you OK?' but they're not over protective. They stand up for me so if anyone ever said anything against me, it would be, 'She's my sister, don't you dare say anything'. Once a girl in my sister's class – her mother is in a wheelchair – and my sister were having a discussion with another girl. The girl actually said that people in wheelchairs have a pointless life. Both my sister and her friend got very angry, and had a right go at this girl. I think the girl wished she'd never spoken to them to begin with.

My being in a wheelchair makes no difference to my close friends. They just like me and treat me as if I wasn't in a wheelchair. There are problems if I want to go to their houses. It is difficult, so I end up not being invited: for example, if they are having a party, and I can't get there because of my wheelchair. Often the parents are less worried than my friends are. But people who don't know me so well are always worried in case they hurt my feelings or somebody else's at the same time. We were doing a drama thing, and I was originally going to have to be a sports teacher, which didn't look right. I was supposed to be teaching a class, and they didn't want to say anything in case they hurt my feelings saying, 'You can't be a sports teacher because you're in a wheelchair'. I didn't want to say anything either in case they'd think I was a bit silly and it ended up that we were both thinking the same thing but didn't want to say anything in case we hurt other people. In the end I became something else and somebody else became the sports teacher.

My teachers don't allow me to use my wheelchair as an excuse, either. I can't say, 'I'm sorry I didn't do my essay because my arms were tired from pushing all day in my wheelchair'. They wouldn't buy that. They would say, 'Don't you dare try and say that'. They don't allow any differences and if I did try, I think I would probably be told off.

The school has done a lot to make things easier for me with my wheelchair. They've put in ramps and lifts. For instance, in my boarding house they had to put a lift in so that I could get up to my bedroom. We all have cubicles which are very tiny, in fact so small that my wheelchair couldn't get into a single one because it was just that little bit too small.

So they knocked two into one and I'm now the envy of the house . I've got the big room and they've put in ramps. So that I can get to my chemistry lessons, they've just bought a sort of chair that walks up the stairs: it's got four wheels, two sets, and they do like a tank thing and walk up the stairs.

And they don't let me off the housework, either. We all have to do it, every day from 8.15 to 8.30 am. This term I've had the toilets as my housework, which I have to sweep and make sure they're all clean. I have to refill hand towels, empty the bins and things like that. The only problem I have come across is sweeping up the dust but I ask somebody else to do that. I'm taking ten subjects at GCSE: two English, Maths, it's compulsory for us to take RE; I am also taking Latin, three Sciences, Drama and IT. I think my favourite subject would have to be Biology or English. I'm not particularly good at English, but I'm getting better, and I like reading anything I can get my hands on. I like books with a twist in them. I hate predictable books, and I get bored by them, but I also like historical books. I think that I would like to do IT, Maths and Biology for A level, and then after that I would like to go to university. I think I'd like to go into law or some sort of medical research.

I don't think they'll have found a way to repair spinal injury in my lifetime but you don't know. I would be extremely happy if they did, but I don't want to think too much about it in case they don't and then I would get a little upset and I don't want to do that. I do think they should try and do everything they possibly can and find some way of curing it because it would be such a help to so many people. It would be such a relief. You wouldn't have to worry about the places your wheelchair is going to have to go in your life – you would just sort of walk away from your wheelchair, wouldn't you?

I don't like doctors. They're not very good at giving you all the information. If you have a problem they either try to put it in such a nice way that you don't understand what they are saying, or they put it very bluntly and you still don't understand what they are saying. I hate going to hospital, partly because I'm not used to being with other disabled people, and people who are sick, and I don't particularly like that.

I have to go in to Stoke Mandeville every year for a week to make sure everything is working. We have a new brace and calliper fitting. I never look forward to that week and as soon as it's over, I'm glad.

One thing that's rather difficult for me is transport. I can't really use public transport unless we are going as a family, then we sometimes take the train to Eastbourne to our friends. I'd never be able to use a train on my own, or a bus, although I've heard that in some parts of the country there are official buses with lifts in. When we do go by rail my Dad has to help me in and out of the train by lifting my chair and me and things. Often train stations don't have lifts, so there's stairs. I once went with my family on the tube. It wasn't much different to the train, but there were escalators which my Dad had to help me down. The lift was permanently broken which is really annoying when you're in a wheelchair, and anyway the doors were a bit too narrow for a wheelchair to get through.

Usually, if I want to go anywhere, I ask my Mum to take me in the car. It means we always have to plan ahead and we can't do things, like going to the cinema, on the spur of the moment. If I do want to go somewhere, it isn't only the transport that's the problem. We once went to an old house, and they refused point-blank to let me in, in case I crashed or damaged anything or I ruined the carpets by wheeling over them. It was not a particularly nice situation, and I think they were being a bit silly because I wouldn't have done any more damage than anyone else. At cinemas and places like that in London, because they're normally buildings where you have to go up steps, they refuse to let me in because of fire regulations. One time my friend and I were going to the cinema and they refused to let me in. A man in the queue said, 'Oh look, I'll take full responsibility for her. I'll make sure she comes out if there's a fire, and if need be I'll carry her'. They still refused to let me in and so in the end we had to go home. You have to pursue them a lot of the time, saying 'Oh, if there's a fire I'll be OK', but because you know they're going to say something, you always look for a place where there are no steps inside, and things like that.

Sometimes, even if people try to help, it's unhelpful. Like my old headmistress at my primary school. She felt it would be useful, whenever I was away, to explain to the school and class how wonderful I was in actually managing to cope. She sort of put me on a pedestal which made things worse, because the class and the other children in the school resented it. It didn't work and actually caused quite a lot more damage. I got a lot of stick for being Miss Goody-Two-Shoes. I can't really say I've had any help that's been a lifeline, everything depends on people's attitudes. I've coped perfectly well emotionally, but then I've never known any different. I try not to make comparisons. I try to look at the more positive things in life. There will always be people who are better than you at some things, but if they are better than me, it's not because they are not in a wheelchair, it's maybe because they're cleverer or something.

There's more awareness now that people with disabilities aren't that different. The biggest difference is that they may not be able to run around, but that's about as far as it goes. But there are still far too many people who say that there is a difference so let's exclude them, but I think that's very wrong and they should definitely do something about it now. Too many buildings, especially in London, are full of steps with very narrow doors which a younger child can get through but an adult couldn't. Generally speaking toilets are not big enough to accommodate wheelchairs. Escalators instead of lifts is again a bit annoying because you can't get down an escalator but you can get down in a lift. A lot of the time lifts are broken.

If they said that you are breaking the law if you do not provide access for wheelchairs, I'm sure that things would improve immediately for us. There would be a few people who would say, 'Oh well, you're costing me money, because I have to make a door wider or put an extra toilet in', but I'm sure there are plenty of other people out there who are saying 'What's the difference?' It isn't fair to discriminate against us, so I think in the future there will be a lot more people on our side.

If they did bring in such a law, I'm sure there would be a lot of people saying 'That's not fair', but eventually they're going to have to provide access for us. So they should do it now rather than in the future.

I think that you have to make people near you aware, and then make the not-so-near people aware, and eventually just make everybody who has anything distantly to do with you or people like you aware that there isn't a difference. I'm sure that if enough people were made aware, pretty soon everybody would realize that there isn't a difference.

My way of dealing with discrimination is to ignore it. If it gets really bad, though, I'll bite back. Sometimes kindness can be extremely embarassing. Once when I was on holiday in Scotland, we were sitting in the hotel quite late in the evening. All of a sudden two old ladies came up and gave me money. They were talking in very thick Scottish accents, saying, 'Isn't she wonderful' and that sort of thing. I was there with my sisters and I didn't understand a word. I was very embarrassed and the ladies were patting me, and I didn't know whether to give it back, because of not wanting to be rude. It was so brilliant in a way – £100!

There are always people who will come up and say, 'How are you doing, dear' or 'Are you coping OK?', and it gets quite embarrassing. I sort of smile and wish they weren't there. As soon as they've said their little bit I sort of try and escape as fast as possible.

My advice to any young person growing up with a spinal injury would be, do what you want to do and ignore other people. If you feel you want to do something, then go ahead and do it, but don't let other people decide for you what you can and can't do. If people are willing to help you, then don't totally ignore them, but if you're wanting desperately to do something and they say that it's not a good idea because of your wheelchair, ignore them. Just go ahead and do it.

I was on a telethon programme once. I was selected through the SIA. The programme was asking for two children and they said 'Yes, you'd be a good person to do it' and that's it. It was only briefly, I was only on for a second.

I was quite relaxed about taking part. I didn't realize that they were going to use it all on television. I saw the television cameras and I thought that was because the Duchess of York was there. I didn't know any more until I was watching television and said, 'Hey, look, there's me!'

I even met the Duchess of York, but she was surrounded by millions of bodyguards, I had one really embarassing moment, though, because there was only one large toilet, and I had to use it because of the wheelchair. It had been reserved for the Duchess of York as her private toilet, but I didn't realize that, and she was actually waiting outside for me to hurry up.

Family holidays, well, I just do what the family does unless they are doing something I can't do. Last summer my parents and sisters went to Spain for a walking holiday and I stayed with friends. I actually preferred staying here because I had lovely hot weather and they had horrible rain in Madrid. I had the better of it that time, but I just normally join in with whatever the family does. Once we get there and if there is a difficulty, we just work out how to overcome it.

One time when the SIA were having a new building opened by Princess Anne, I gave flowers to her. My photo was in the newspaper. I was very little, I would have been six and I remember I was wearing my favourite dress and I was wonderfully pleased to be giving flowers to somebody. Also, I was in a local magazine for playing my violin with some friends to raise some money.

I've been playing the violin for ten years and so you would think that I might be good, but I'm actually very bad, I'm only on grade three. I'm not very musically minded, but I try to strum along. My sisters play the violin and cello. I used to play in an orchestra but I had to give it up because I found I'd got too much school work. I like all sorts of music, though I prefer playing classical music to listening to it. I don't particularly have a favourite composer, or a favourite pop group at the moment either – I just like bits of songs. I don't have any other hobbies, but I read all sorts of magazines, especially those for teenagers, like *Just Seventeen.*

Mike Marten

Mike Marten was born in 1958 and joined the Royal Navy in 1977, becoming a diver. He sustained his spinal cord injury in a water-ski-ing accident while on a NATO exercise in France in 1987. He was discharged from the Royal Navy in 1989. He lives in Fareham, near Portsmouth. Divorced in 1991, he has no children.

I spent ten active years in the Navy. I was taking part in a NATO exercise in the South of France in June 1987 and, on a day off midway through the exercise, decided to try water ski-ing. I was pulled over into shallow water and hit my head on the seabed. The impact was enough to break my neck. I spent a week in France and then was flown back to England where I went to Odstock Hospital in Salisbury, Wiltshire, because that was the nearest geographically to where I lived.

I spent the following year in Odstock. It's actually a superb unit, and I'm very glad that I went there as opposed to Stoke Mandeville. When I came out, my wife and I had to find a new place to live because our house just wasn't suitable. We'd only moved in three weeks before the accident, but it was modern, not suitable for adaptation. My wife found a bungalow which we subsequently bought, and I moved into a Naval hospital while it was adapted. It was gutted, completely renovated inside and then we moved in. I then spent a few months at home before going down to Exeter to St Loye's College, a training college for the disabled. It trains disabled people from all walks of life and with all disabilities for commerce and industry. I did a commercial skills course which included word-processing, accounts, book-keeping, computer literacy and that kind of thing, which I found quite hard at the time. I pride myself on getting high exam results and that all went well, but while I was staying there my wife Jane had an opportunity actually to sit down and realize what had happened to her life as well as what had happened to mine. The realities of it all came up and hit her, knocked her off her feet, and she had to take six weeks off work. She went and lived with her Mum and Dad for that time, was in floods of tears every night, and went through a deep depression. When I came back from St Loye's we tried to get our marriage back together, going to marriage guidance and so on, but it just didn't work. We eventually got divorced. The goal posts basically had been moved, and Jane wasn't happy with the situation. I'm still very good friends with her; she's since re-married and hopefully now is very happy.

About that time, in 1991, I was invited to go out to America with some ex-servicemen I'd never heard of, and had an absolutely superb time – socializing, getting drunk, eating far too much and occasionally pushing round the track in my wheelchair pretending to be an athlete. Since then I've got more and more involved in athletics, keeping fit and training hard, and so that takes up quite a large part of my time. Inevitably I find that I'm more involved, and have been invited to sit on more and more disability committees and consultation groups. It's got to such a point now that I've actually started to turn people down because I don't want my whole life to revolve around disability issues. I'm very busy, and involved with four or five important groups, but I've drawn a line, and so I suppose that almost brings us up to the present day.

If you want a character assessment, I reckon I'm a reasonably easy-going chap, and there's nothing I like more than enjoying myself, socializing. I can be fiercely determined and tenacious if I decide something's right or something is mine, and if I really want something, then it's going to take a lot to stop me. It's an attitude which I think came from being a Royal Navy diver, the attitude where if there's a job on, you've got to get out there and do it, you can't say 'I'm sorry I can't'. This stands me in good stead now because if I want to go on holiday, if I want to do a particular sport or activity, or if I want to go anywhere, it can be organized. It may not be that easy, but it can be organized, so that's the sort of person I am – I don't think too much about the problems, I just know that when I get there I will cope with it.

My father was in the Navy. When we were young, we'd gather round the Sunday lunch table and he'd spin us his lies and exaggerations which of course we fell for, being kids. So really from my earliest days I'd decided that I wanted to follow my Dad into the Navy. He was one of the first divers that went through when they first started the diving branch, and so I decided I wanted to follow on. The diving branch is different from any other branch in the Navy for several reasons, but mainly because the work is very exciting and fulfilling. I was immensely proud to be a diver. It's always challenging because you're working in an alien environment – humans aren't designed to be underwater – so you have to control yourself, and remain calm. When it goes pitch black, you're underneath a pontoon, and you don't know what way's up, down or out, you've got to remain in control of yourself, so it's a demanding job. We didn't travel that much as a rule, because most of the diving work we did was around the UK – servicing our ships, working on ship's bottoms, locating and investigating objects on seabeds and so on. Having said that, though, there were several really notable jobs that I was lucky enough to be involved in, particularly in my last year in the Navy. One of them was out in the United Arab Emirates. A super-tanker was hit by a missile fired from an Iraqi helicopter, and so a team of five of us flew out there for a week. We spent a day and a half on board a super-tanker getting rid of an unexploded missile which was lodged in the engine room. That was an absolutely fantastic job, one highly cherished by all divers, as they all wanted to be on a Gulf job.

In the early part of 1987, there was the Zeebrugge ferry disaster, and I was involved in that. I was part of a diving team at the time called the Fleet Clearance Diving Team. They had worldwide commitments: any job anywhere in the world that involved British naval interest or British interest, we were sent to deal with, hence the Iraqi job. On the night that the *Herald of Free Enterprise* went down, I wasn't contacted because I was as drunk as a skunk in an Indian restaurant with some friends. However, when I woke up the next day, and saw it on the news, I rang in and was told that the last thing they wanted at the time was divers. A month or so later, they started to get the ship upright, and then they needed to get the bodies off. That's when I became involved there, on the body recovery phase. It was hard work. As you walked down one side of the ship, from the ceiling at an angle down to the floor was just a mass of arms, legs, bodies, blankets, furniture, tables, all packed in deep mud. On the other uppermost side of the ship it was absolutely clean and in pristine condition because it had been washed constantly by the sea. Our job was to dig each person out by hand, drag them to a central point and get them put in bags and trays, and then shipped off. All seven of us were proud to be there. I don't think any of us thought twice about it, we just got stuck in. I can well remember coming home and my neighbours said. 'Oh I couldn't do that job, I don't know how you do it'.

I've got a broken neck at level C6/C7 – the C stands for cervical. I'm paralysed from about nipple-line downwards, with no function in my hands, but over a period of years I've learnt to adapt and use a lot of tricks. On top of that bowels, bladder and sex organs are all very badly affected – they don't work. That's something in common with 99 percent of all spinal cord injuries, because the nerves that control those three very important parts of your life are right down low and they are nearly always affected.

It was very interesting that as soon as I had my accident, I knew I'd broken my neck. The second I hit my head on the seabed I knew that my neck was broken. When my mates came out to me and towed me back to the jetty I was moaning that I'd broken my neck and that I was going to be paralysed, yet within half an hour my mind had submerged all that, it was obviously too painful to live with. For the next three months I buried it deep and then what had happened gradually started to seep through. I'd been forced to lie in bed for that period, so the enforced inactivity was starting to crack me up. One night at about two in the morning, I asked them to take me out and I just screamed my head off in another room, just crying and blaming every bastard, every God, all the things under the sun. That heralded three or four months of very severe depression. Most days in hospital they would have to pick me up and put me into a wheelchair because I was very weak, and would faint if I had the slightest bout of exertion. The major thing that hurt was the loss of pride – from being fit, strong, and indestructible to being someone who couldn't comb his hair because his arms ached, who couldn't push a wheelchair ten yards without stopping and feeling dizzy. So almost every day I would have to go into a room on my own and just sit and cry. I remember saying to my wife, 'I feel like there's been some mistake because I wasn't put on this earth to be quadraplegic'.

Gradually that crying each day became crying every other day and then every two or three days. A couple of important things helped me come to terms with the emotional side of it. First, two of my mates came up to the hospital and took me out. We went down the pub and had a really good time. Next morning, when you've had a real good time the night before, it's hard to wake up and say, 'I really enjoyed last night, I had a great time, but I want to die because I'm so fed up'. What you actually do is you say, 'I can't wait to do that again'. That's the secret, looking forward to the next time, and that's what you need. So that was important, as were two unrelated accidents in America where people were killed. Some eighteen people in a mini-van, including young children, were killed on the way back from church. Many more were wiped out in a plane crash off Washington Bridge. You just suddenly think, I'm blaming God for my accident, what about all these people? All these people with bad luck and all blaming God, it can't be all his fault. I'm not religious anyway, but I realized I had to blame someone, even though it was just an accident. It's just part of life, and once you accept that, you can accept a whole load more in your life as well.

That attitude helped to carry me through, although that wasn't the end of the story, but those were two significant and helpful points that started me on the road to rehabilitation. Thereafter it was just a matter of time really. I noticed that I would cry, and be desperately upset, and then I wouldn't cry for three months. In that three months in between I'd be okay, and then I wouldn't cry for five months, seven months, then a year, then two years. All of a sudden I'd wonder when was the last time I'd cried because of the accident, and now I can't think when the last time was. I'm much more fatalistic now than I was before my accident. I just know that things happen in life and that you haven't got any control over them. I know that we're all going to die one day and I'm prepared to part with all my family eventually. Hopefully I'll understand that it's just part of life in the same way that I've had to accept my accident. All of my life before the accident was devoted to keeping fit, looking after my body and being strong: I'd started boxing at the age of ten and had over 100 amateur fights, and my idea of enjoyment was running ten miles and then doing a hundred press-ups. All that was taken away from me, and suddenly I felt, 'Well, hang on, let's not get too bound up with my own issues', so it's put things in perspective.

The most positive aspect is all the fantastic people I've met, all the nice people I meet day in, day out. When I am in my car I need someone to get the chair out of the boot for me so that I can get out of the car; likewise when I get into the car I need someone to put the chair in the back. I'll just pull up in a car park and ask a total stranger to do that for me, and I've never met anyone who'd even think twice about helping me out. The public are fantastic, always polite. When you are independent, you are insular, and you can cope; when you need help, as I do now, you find there are people there. I've got fantastic neighbours as well, really good friends, and every day I meet kindness which I wouldn't have met before because I wouldn't have needed it. That's very positive, you know.

In many instances, when I'm dealing with other people, my disability gives me an advantage, a head start almost. When I go bounding into a building, and I say, 'Hi, I'm Mike Marten, I'm here to see so-and-so', people can be taken aback, or can be wrong-footed. They don't quite know how to deal with this chap in a chair. I spent twenty-seven years walking round and dealing with Joe Public, and you are nothing strange to me; but I'm a bit strange to you, so immediately I can be in control because I'm at ease and I know what's happening whereas others are a little bit uneasy.

I like sporting activities very much. I like any kind of challenge whether it be physical endurance or whatever, anything that I think I can try, that's what I find very satisfying. I'm not quite sure why, I don't know if I'm trying to prove it to other people or to myself. I'm just enjoying pushing myself, not as hard as I can, but pretty hard. The first time I did a half marathon I'd done absolutely no training for it whatsoever. I had one week's notice and I had an ordinary everyday wheelchair which had to be pushed manually, and my girlfriend at the time who I felt a great deal for, said, 'There's absolutely no way in the world you can do it'. So just out of bloody mindedness, I pushed the thirteen miles. It took me six hours, and I was not only last but the person who was second to last was three hours ahead of me. That was 1992. I did the half marathon again a year later in the same chair, and it took me five and a half hours. Then I did it the year after that in a racing chair and it only took me one hour, twenty-six minutes, so that's the difference the racing chair makes. Instead of being last on both occasions out of 4,000, I beat 3,500 of them, so that was good. The Berlin marathon, which was my first full marathon, I did in two hours, forty-six minutes, and that's a really good course. I did the London and then a week after that I did a second marathon on the South coast.

Sky-diving, again I've done that three times, and that was very satisfying and exciting. I like to raise a bit of money for charity by doing it every couple of years if I can. The way it works is, you're strapped to the chest of another man and the pair of you come out of a plane at 11,000 feet, tumble for about 6,000 feet then come down together under the parachute. Hopefully there's a catching party on the ground, and with these big, highly manoeuvrable parachutes you should come in to a fairly safe landing. It doesn't always work that way, though, and in fact in the three that I've done, only one did work that way. The other two have been quite rough landings.

I was always interested in physical training, just being in a gym, just keeping fit and looking after my body. When I had my accident, training almost went out of the window really, but then I started having weights bandaged into my hands so I could sit in my chair and do a little bit. The progression to being a serious athlete, which I almost am, started off in America, pushing round a track in an ordinary chair when others were in racing chairs and thrashing you. I didn't care, because I was only out there for the social side of it, but then I began thinking, well, how can I do this a bit better? It was a gradual progression to taking sport more and more seriously. The other two sports I do are table tennis and archery, and of my three sports, table tennis is probably my greatest love, I really enjoy it: the bat is taped into my hand and I'll play for hours. Archery is not a great passion but if I'm ever going to be picked for a disabled team, it will probably be an archery team because I'm quite good at that for my level of injury. Again the bow is bandaged into my hand, and I have a hook device to pull the string back with. Racing is another sport that I really enjoy because it allows me to work hard physically and keep fit and strong. I'm a very competitive bloke, but I always compete against myself. I'll get in a race and I'll push as hard and as fast as I can. If perchance that's harder and faster than the other guys, then that's wonderful, but I don't think it ever will be, it never has been to date. I'm just a realist, and really I'm enjoying pushing myself to a large extent.

My brother, Anthony, who is perfectly able-bodied, and I are very competitive. He races while I push, and we try to beat each other. It's wonderful to be able to ring him up and gloat that I beat him in a race. I stuffed him in the Berlin Marathon! The first race he won by about two minutes and neither of us were fit – that was only a 10 kilometre race at Gosport. Then we entered the Brighton/Hove half-marathon and I got a bad puncture. I wasted an hour and a half trying to replace the wheel and eventually I had to withdraw because I wasn't going anywhere after that time. I compete with him at table tennis as well. Months or years ago when I was in Odstock, I was so weak I couldn't push a wheelchair anywhere, and yet here I am ringing my brother up badgering him to challenge me in a race, that's great. That competitive edge is something I never thought I'd get again against my brother.

I don't think anyone without a real experience of disability understands the effect of lack of bladder and bowel control on your life. I mean, there's nothing quite like pushing round Sainsbury's to get your shopping, and piddling yourself. You then have to make a decision, 'Right, am I going to stop everything now, and go out all embarrassed, or am I going to carry on shopping?' After a period of time I decided that when that happened I'd put a bag over my lap and carry on shopping because that's what I was there for. People are very good in the way that they try and cope with it, particularly older people, or people who have had children and are well used to dirty nappies, but it's a major complication, it's a consideration.

I don't think I associate it with my childhood, because it's only as a result of my injury that my bladder is no longer under control, so there's nothing I can do about it. It is embarrassing because I'll be sitting there with my lap full of piddle or my pants full of something else. But after a time I started to understand that there was nothing I could do about it. It wasn't my fault. All that's required is someone willing to help get it sorted out. It's an inconvenience now, whereas at first I found it quite unpleasant, and I would come back home and have a good cry from embarrassment. Incontinence takes a lot of thinking about sometimes: you know, if I go there and get caught short, and I can't get to a loo, what am I going to do?

A lot of people either do an inordinate amount of planning to make things secure, or they don't go anywhere – a lot of people daren't leave their homes. I won't do either of those things, I just go and cope with whatever happens, even if it means asking someone where the local hospital is, and going there for help. If I'm going to go somewhere on a regular basis, like to my girlfriend's house in Evesham, then I'll start to make a few proper enquiries. I contacted the surgery in Evesham and told them of my disability and asked if ever I needed help, could I call on them? 'Please do, Mr Marten,' they said 'That's no problem, you're more than welcome.' That's established now, and no problem, but if I'm going somewhere as a one-off, I just cope with the situation if it goes wrong when I get there.

When I was still in hospital and got a full bowel, I would have to call the nurses and wait hours for them to come and give me what is known as a manual evacuation, where they literally help it out. Well in that time my blood pressure would be going up, I'd be sweating, I'd be intensely uncomfortable, and obviously my underpants would be full of everything. I suddenly started to wonder what I could do about it. Now I've got a shower chair in my room, I just position it alongside the bed, transfer on to the other side of the bed and get over, get myself undressed and on to the shower chair. I then just trundle over to the loo and deal with it in nature's most normal way. It's a fantastic development and now it's escalated. If I went on holiday with someone in the past, they would have to be taught how to do a manual to help which obviously not everyone was going to be willing to do. Now all we do is transfer – I can pretty well transfer on my own on to the loo – and take care of it that way, so that is a great release, a major step forward in my life. It may be unusual but now I'm doing the most basic function very nearly in the ordinary way.

I think it's vitally important for people to understand that people in wheelchairs, almost regardless of their disability, do have a sexual aspect to their characters. Just as earlier on I identified the most positive aspect of my disability as being the wonderful people I've met, undoubtedly the worst thing for me is the catastrophic effect that the accident's had on my sex life. I have no feeling from my chest down, and that obviously includes the genital area. I also can't climax, so having children is very difficult, but by no means impossible. I've also lost that glorious feeling of orgasm, as well as the ability to move and take an active role with a partner. These are all significant problems, and this aspect of disability is one that is very rarely discussed. Nevertheless all disabled people have got a sexual side to their nature.

I've got a lovely girlfriend now, and we've got a very active sex life, but what I'm having trouble with, even though it's nearly seven years since my accident, is perfecting and maintaining an erection. I've tried all sorts of things but this is still something that isn't perfectly sorted out. The beautiful thing about a neck break as opposed to a back break is that you normally retain the ability to get a reflex erection, whereas with a back break you go permanently flaccid. I can get the erection, but it cannot be maintained long enough for sexual intercourse. That of course is coupled with the lack of bladder control, which means that even if I can maintain the erection I might well be piddling anyway. Other guys in my position will have sorted this out years ago, and they'll be wondering what I'm going on about, but I've just found it difficult to find and try the various types of equipment, the various injections and devices you can use.

I can't say that I come across a lot of discrimination, but possibly if I was applying for jobs and being turned down simply because I was in a wheelchair, I'd start to get pretty cheesed off about it. I don't really think a great deal about discrimination, I just get on with my life, but obviously there is a degree of discrimination against us in as much as public transport isn't fully public, for instance. Trains aren't fully accessible and you might have to sit in a guard's van, or you might have to ring up twenty-four hours before you want to go anywhere. Lots of buildings have just a few steps, which means I cannot get in. Of course, having said that, I will get in because I'll get passers-by to help me up the steps, but I can't get in easily on my own. Other people may want to visit that building but be less determined, so will be put off. Society is disabling us and fighting against us in a way. Things are improving without a doubt, and in general I haven't found the attitude of individuals to be discriminatory.

I suppose I'm not too hot on personal relationships, because I'm divorced. That was almost to be expected, for two reasons really. First, both my wife and I were in the services. Then, when we had to leave, we were suddenly spending a lot of time with each other, which we weren't used to. We both started feeling, 'For Christ's sake, you get right under my bloody feet, you do'. A lot of services marriages break up for the same reason. The second factor in the break-up of my marriage was, of course, the disability. Again you can expect marriages to break up, because the goal posts have been moved so dramatically. But if you combine the two, you leave the Navy, you're spending all your time with somebody, and then you've got a major disability, it's a recipe for disaster. So to an extent I can certainly understand why Jane left, and I think part of the mistake there was that she became so involved with my care. She was such a conscientious person and she did become more of a carer than a wife. I started wanting to shrug off the lessons of Odstock and say, 'Listen, I want to challenge this, I want to be a bit daring', whereas Jane would still be thinking of all the things she'd learned about how to look after me – I've got to make sure the sheets are tight so that he doesn't get pressure sores, I've got to make sure he doesn't do this, doesn't do that . . . . She was helping with bowel care as well, and I realize now that was a mistake. I make quite sure that Emma, my present girlfriend, is involved as little as possible. I try really hard to dress myself, but I do find that with hand function gone, pulling on socks and trousers when I'm lying on the bed is quite hard work.

My parents were very deeply shocked by my accident, and the whole family was very sad at first, although that was never transmitted to me when they came to visit. They were very cheerful, very bright, but obviously when you hear that your son has broken his neck, you are going to be shocked. I think most of my family admire me now for the way that I've got on. Again they don't particularly let that show, except for my Mum. My brothers just take the mickey out of me as they've always done. There isn't an attitude of 'let's spare his feelings'. My disability is totally disregarded now.

Most of my friends have been fantastic. I've got several very good friends, ex-Royal Navy divers, who have stuck with me through thick and thin. There are many guys out there doing their various jobs and I might see them maybe once a year. They might say, 'Look, sorry, I haven't written to you, I am sorry, mate,' and I say, 'Well, I haven't written to you, have I?' It's a two-edged thing. In the Navy and the services, serving with someone for a year and a half, you become really good friends and then you might not see them for five years. You don't write to each other because it just isn't something that guys in the services normally do, so I've got no axe to grind if I don't hear from most of them. What I do know is that if they're in town or if we get together one evening, we'll have a damn good thrash!

I don't know how I'd cope if I couldn't drive. I love it and it's an absolute lifeline to me. Public transport is no big hobby horse for me because I can drive. I'm doing over 20,000 miles a year driving around, visiting people, so that's something that's vitally important to me.

After I'd finished at St Loye's (the training college) I wasn't really looking for work because it was at that time that Jane had her depression. I did get involved with a charity in Portsmouth called DIAL (Disability Information Advice Line) and I used to produce a newsletter for them because of the new commercial skills I'd learnt – the word processing, desktop publishing and so on. I've been getting more and more into charity work since then, but I haven't had any paid employment as such. After my accident, the Navy retained me on full pay for two years. That was a tremendous help because I had no financial worries. I do also want to mention the fund-raising that my diving mates did for me after my accident. There were guys all over the world jumping into swimming pools, jumping off boats, running and all sorts and they raised £16,000 for me which was a fantastic amount. They just were absolutely superb.

I now get what's termed a war pension because the Navy were implicated in my accident. I also get a couple of State benefits, attendance allowance and mobility allowance which I've traded in for my car, but then the rest is made up as a result of the war pension. Amazingly that all went fairly smoothly. Servicemen can experience difficulty because they're suddenly kicked out of the services system then they're not really in the civilian system either. I was lucky, I had a very good chap who helped me. I don't know off the top of my head what the exact figures are, but I get mobility allowance, attendance allowance and invalidity benefit. I also get my war pension and my Navy pension. Then there are things that they call comfort allowances. Of course, I do have additional costs, I've got this electric chair which cost me £600 to buy, and I just had to replace the batteries which were £100. My tyres are £26 a pair and they wear out. My car cost £1,300 extra on top to get it adapted.

I feel that I've got to speak out for those who are perhaps getting very little. Other disabled people have got a much sharper view of it than I have, but there ought to be some other benefit called disability income, or something like that, which really tries to take into account the additional costs. I've outlined some already, but because of my double incontinence, my washing machine and tumble dryer are always on; because I'm pushing my wheelchair all the time, the cuffs of my shirts get dirty and worn. There are lots of costs that you very rarely think of: for instance, a lot of people have dietary problems, so their foods might need to be fresh or have to be of a certain type. There should be a system that will give you an allowance for these indirect additional costs.

My health is very good as a rule and so I have very few reasons to go and see doctors, but I do have a very good doctor locally. I've built up a rapport with her and so now when I need more equipment or whatever I just send in for a repeat prescription so there's no grilling about why I want something. She's very trustworthy and she knows I'm trustworthy, so I get on very well with her. There have been various times when I've needed help from doctors, and I've never found them wanting in any way. Having said that, though, if I had an accident, like being involved in a car crash or something, I would be dubious about going to a National Health Service hospital simply because I know that so many people end up back at spinal units to deal with pressure sores they've picked up from treatment in an NHS hospital. They just don't seem to be tuned in to the needs for turning and the extra problems of a paralysed spinally injured person. I've never had pressure sores, but I'm very lucky as I've got the skin of a rhino. I've slept in the back of mini vans, I've slept on settees, I've been drunk and slept on the floor, and I always get away with it.

At first I needed a great deal of help with basic things like getting up and dressed in the morning, particularly when the house wasn't adapted. Having the house adapted is vital because if I can't get to the kettle, I can't even make myself a cup of tea; if I can't reach the taps, I can't even have a drink; if the bread's up out of my way I can't make a sandwich. If things are where you can reach them then you can do so much more for yourself. Because I'm incontinent, I wear a bag on my leg; before the house was adapted, I couldn't get to the toilet to empty that so someone had to come in and do that. Someone had to help me into bed at night and so there was lots of support and lots of help needed, but gradually as the house was adapted, I developed, trying new methods of doing things, so the level of help required and given gradually dropped off.

I am actually going to have an operation at the end of October or November sometime, on my hands, because of the lack of movement. It's a tendon transplant, which is quite commonplace in Australia and America, but isn't done very often over here. They are going to start doing them in Odstock Hospital and the idea is to relocate a couple of tendons in my arm to give me a very basic hand-open, hand-close function. I won't be able to play the piano, but then I couldn't before the accident, so that's no problem! But it will enable me, for instance, to open my hand, close it and get a good grip.

With regards to research into spinal cord injury, I don't feel that there will ever be any research done or breakthroughs made that will be of real benefit to me. Just say, for example, that right now there was a marvellous operation, a piece of computer gadgetry that could bypass the damaged cords and make me better, where would I be in the queue? If there are, say, 300 people a year who have spinal cord injuries in this country, and it's seven years since I had my injury, where am I in that queue? What about all the people before me? I just accept that this is how I am and I am this way for life and get on with it. Thank God for spinal cord research, let them find something so that when the young guys of tomorrow injure themselves we can get them up and out again. My Mum will always say, 'Mike, you never know what's round the corner,' so she might need to hang on to that hope, but I can see the reality behind it. Even if there was this miracle cure, my bowels and my bladder haven't worked for seven years, how are they going to react? What about my muscles and my legs and my stomach, they've not exercised for seven years, so they're not just going to flash up and work again.

I can remember a conversation I had with the consultant when I was in Odstock. He thought that in the future, at the scene of an accident where someone has a spinal cord injury, they would do one of two things: they would either freeze the spinal cord which would prevent it swelling, because it's the swelling within the backbone that often causes the damage; or they would actually open up the backbone and allow the swelling to occur naturally and then subside. I don't know what's been done since then, how far advanced it all is, but both of these seem perfectly feasible to me.

Odstock Hospital was absolutely superb. It had only been open two years, it was bright and modern and the staff were fantastic. It was a forward-thinking hospital and I'm very glad I went there.

One thing Odstock didn't do was to help me with the psychological effects of my injury. I can remember really wanting to die at various stages, just being so desperately unhappy. The problem is that you're there for a year, so you get to know people very well, the patients and staff, and they're used to seeing this happy smiling chap. With all the banter that goes on in these hospitals, it's very hard then to open up and say, 'I'm desperately unhappy', even though everyone knows that you must be. What is required, I think, is a weekly routine visit to a psychologist or counsellor, someone detached from the unit that you're not going to see every day. It needs to happen routinely because that allows you to put on the bravado, 'Oh, bloody hell, I've got that appointment on Wednesday, what a waste of space', but you can then go there, make use of it, then come back and maintain that bravado. I wasn't offered anything like that.

I think some degree of depression is inevitable. How severe it is will depend on the sort of person you are, your history and your background. I did meet one chap in hospital who assured me absolutely categorically that he was depressed for one hour and that was it, after that he just cracked on and totally disregarded it, I've known other people who just take years and years, and quite honestly I look upon them as miserable bastards. Even though what has happened to them is terrible, I can't help thinking, 'For Christ's sake, crack out of it'. When Jane was with me and very unhappy I'd say to her, 'I understand what's happened, Jane, but look at where we live, it's a nice bright house, I've got a good pension, you've got a job, we've both got cars. Let's be thankful we're not in some damp council house with no money and no prospects.' Now my problem is frustration with myself for not being able to do simple things as efficiently as I used to be able to. If I want to pick up four or five things and take them somewhere, the only way is on my lap. I'll pile it all up, then go to move the wheels and one falls off. As I lean down, another falls off, and I can't then pick them up, and I start getting annoyed. These frustrations have come upon me since the accident, whereas when I was fit and in the Navy I didn't have them at all.

I'd never been temped to try fringe treatments, but Jane was prepared to try anything. When I was coming out of hospital for weekends, Jane was obviously desperate to get me better, desperate to get me back to the person that she had married and she organized a faith healer to come and visit. I had absolutely no faith in this chap whatsoever, but I recognized very quickly that I was in a no-win situation: if I just dismissed him and said, 'Look, the guy's a jerk', then Jane could say to me sometime, 'Well, the only reason you're still in your chair is because you wouldn't listen to that chap, it's your own fault.' He did come round and there was like this laying on of hands and all this sort of hogwash, and I had to close my eyes and put up with it. But eventually, after about three or four weeks, the chap turned up and I said, 'Listen, I've put up with it, I've not believed it for one second, and thank you for your help, but please don't come again.' That was the only alternative medicine that I've been involved in, and I'm not really in any hurry to get involved again, because I found it quite embarrassing.

I have someone who comes in and helps me get dressed each morning, and she comes back twice a week to help with the housework. Margaret's a super lady, I'm very lucky with her, and she doesn't just do housework, she'll put the photos up. Now that wouldn't be in her contract, to put photos up like that, but she is my arms and legs that I can't use, and so she's that flexible, and she's very good. I mentioned that I try and keep Emma away from anything to do with care. As a result, when we are together, I make a real effort to dress myself and to do as much as possible for myself. I know that there are guys out there with injuries very similar to mine, some even worse, who dress themselves routinely every day, or do their own housework. Well, that's good, I respect them for that but the reason I accept help is that I've got lots of other things I want to do with my life. While they're still getting dressed, I'll be fifteen miles up the road on my way somewhere. I've got many more things to worry about than this little bit of independence. I accept that help so that I can get on with my life in other areas, which to me is far more important than just struggling to get dressed every morning. I like to look reasonable and Margaret makes sure that in the morning I'm tucked in, my buttons are done up, and I'm happy then for the day. If I were doing it myself, it might not all be as tucked in as it could be.

Most people think I cope pretty well really. In the spinal units they think I cope pretty well as well. If you've got 100 spinally injured guys with neck breaks, I would say I'm in the top third. I reckon there are two-thirds of people below me that do bugger all, and haven't got half the things going on in their life that I have, and don't have half as much fun. They wouldn't dream of going to Malta with their girlfriend, of just packing up and going, and they wouldn't drive 20,000 miles, and wouldn't do half the things I do. But I'm also well aware that there are guys better than me out there.

I think the support in the house must come into it. Margaret coming in and helping me get dressed each day, helping me with my bowel function and helping me with the housework is very important to me. I know it looks a bit shabby at the moment, but having a nice place where people can come, and I can be proud to bring them, is very important to me.

I find some people's offers to help rather patronizing. I was in Sainsbury's only yesterday and had a fair bit of shopping. I was just starting to put it in the bag at the end of the till, and a lady leaned over and said, 'Here, dear,' and started to do it all for me. She didn't consult me, she didn't ask me, and I had to bite my tongue because I knew that underneath she was trying to be a good person, she was trying to help, but by God she pissed me off. It would have been very easy to have said 'Look, who the hell do you think you are?' but then she'd have gone away thinking she'd never help a disabled person again. That would have been counterproductive, and I certainly wouldn't have felt good.

Mainly, though, I just encounter kindness. People look at you with respect or sympathy, I don't really know which. I was at Blackpool just a few days ago, and I was pushing home along the sea front at midnight. The number of people that came by and just said, 'Evening, mate,' and 'Hi, how are you doing, cold night'. They all just wanted to give me a word of kindness. That's the sort of attitude that I see time and time again, that and the willingness to help.

I think I am changing attitudes in my own way by getting people to help me get my chair in and out of the boot of the car. Other disabled guys can probably get their own chair in and out, and now I'm sure that if I really struggled, if I really thought and thought, and had various things done, I could do it myself too. But the way I see it is that every single time I ask someone to help me, it means they've had a good experience with someone in a wheelchair. Because they've helped a bit, they walk away, nearly always sticking their chest out, and they're chuffed: it all means that I'm constantly meeting the public, and that there are more people having a chat with someone in a wheelchair.

I'm also part of the Spinal Injuries Association's awareness and prevention campaign. It's been going now for probably four or five years. I give talks to schools and colleges on spinal cord injury, and I've spoken to thousands and thousands of schoolchildren. I go on my own now because I've been doing it for several years, or with Lucy Graham from the Spinal Injury Association. Basically we talk about the make-up of the spinal cord and the backbones, how you damage them, how you avoid damaging them. I promote awareness just by being totally honest and open if someone asks a question and not dodging the issue. For instance, I can introduce them to some of the concepts that involve discrimination. I say to them, 'If I was designing this classroom, how high has the ceiling got to be?' and I put my hand up there, as high as it will go, in my wheelchair. I then say, 'Well, what are you people going to do, you'll be all bent over like this'. They would then say, 'Well, Mike, it's all right for you, but we'd get neckache and backache', and I say, 'Well, I'm sorry, I've designed it, and I didn't think about you.' That makes them realize that when someone designs something, they've just got to consider whether every single person can use it.

If I could give one piece of advice to all the other people in my position, I'd say get your immediate surroundings sorted out, so that you can do as much for yourself as you want. Get very busy, get very actively involved in anything and everything that might be going, so that you're out of the house and meeting people. I personally would say don't stick with disabled clubs or disability issues, but if you want to, fine, do whatever makes you feel good. I just feel I don't want to be sucked down into a ever-decreasing circle of disability issues. Get out, live your life, keep busy and keep a smile on your face, and you'll find that there are so many nice people out there. Try with all the strength you've got not to develop a chip on your shoulder and to feel that you've been slighted by this world. It's just part of your life, and the sooner you can accept that, you can carry on enjoying the rest.

I enjoy holidays very much. I've been to America four or five times since my accident at least. In August, I was out in San Antonio, Texas. I'll be going to Malta in about a week or so with my girlfriend, and possibly at the end of July we might go to America as well for a wedding. We flew out to Spain for a few days a while ago just for a little mini break, so I very much enjoy getting abroad. I love France and try to speak the language: Emma enjoys taking the mickey out of me about that, because she's much better than me. Now that I've sorted out my personal little calls of nature, there's really no reason why I can't go anywhere with almost anyone.

I'm thirty-five coming on thirty-six and when I was married my wife and I didn't particularly want children, we just weren't quite ready. I don't know now whether I'm almost getting too old to think about children. It wouldn't happen for about another four or five years at least, and by then I'd be looking at having my first child at forty. It might be an awful strain at sixty, with some twenty-year-old romping around the house and bringing his girlfriends back. As regards the feasibility of it, whilst it's unlikely that it could be done just by intercourse – although that isn't impossible so long as you can maintain the erection – there is the possibility that some semen would be enough to impregnate the woman. You can also go to a spinal unit or to Odstock hospital and they can cause an ejaculation via some kind of stimulator; the woman can then inject the semen via a syringe directly into herself. Alternatively they can put electrodes up your backside and cause an erection and ejaculation that way, which doesn't sound too hot, does it? It most certainly isn't impossible, but at the same time it would be something that needs a fair bit of planning, I would think. Whether it will ever happen, I don't actually know, but really having children is no big burning desire.

I met my current girlfriend, Emma, a year ago in Bournemouth at a Royal British Legion Conference. I was then representing British ex-servicemen who do sports. Emma was there undertaking one of her hobbies, which is standard bearing, so she marches around carrying the standard. We met, obviously we were attracted to each other, swapped addresses, got in contact and we've been together ever since. She is a manager at an AA insurance shop in Swindon. She's perfectly able-bodied.

The one thing I've quite definitely found is that, from a male point of view, the wheelchair is no barrier to meeting the opposite sex and getting girlfriends. I'm no stud, as I've testified earlier, but I've certainly had no trouble at all in getting girlfriends. When one relationship finishes, there's no problem in getting another girlfriend. I think it's different for women in chairs, men seem to be far more reluctant to get involved, but for blokes in chairs, so long as you keep a smile on your face, keep yourself looking reasonable and you're out and about, there are plenty of people who are quite willing to go out with you.

The wheelchair certainly didn't seem to put Emma off. I was sitting there and she came by. We made eye contact and were attracted, you can just tell, so she saw me in the wheelchair on that first day. What did come into it, of course, as we got more intimate in time, were things like the leg bag that I have to wear to hold my urine in. That was something that Emma found quite hard to cope with, so she gave it a nickname. She calls it 'weekly shopping', and the reason why baffles me a bit. At night I connect up a night bag which is a larger version of this, and I piddle from one into the other. The night bag is called 'monthly shopping'. I said something like 'Bloody beef burgers' – just cracked a joke and she said, 'Oh, is that your monthly shopping you've got down there?'

I can remember when I met Emma that I had this fairly blasé attitude, that anyone who meets me must just take me as they find me, this is what I am now and you just have to accept me as I am. But Emma still has a lot to come to terms with; she's only twenty-four and her world was perfect – well, everything in it ought to be perfect. All of a sudden there's me, with so many physical problems and bits hanging on that it takes a lot of getting used to. I've learned a lot from this relationship myself, in as much as it isn't just a case of you see is what you get, this is it, and take me as you find me. I've realized there is a lot to get used to, and Emma has done really well coping with it all.

Judith Jesky

Born in 1956, Judith Jesky is a local government officer for Cambridge City Council. She sustained spinal cord injury in 1969 in a car accident. She lives in Suffolk with her husband.

I had a car accident when I was thirteen years old, and broke my neck at C5/6. First of all, I was admitted to a village hospital, and was later transferred to Lodge Moor Hospital near Sheffield. I think it happened in the July, and I was sent home at about Christmas, so spent about six months in hospital. I was at home for about three months. The headmistress from a special school came to see me there and said she was quite happy to take me, but that I had to go to a rehabilitation unit first. So I went to Mary Marlborough Lodge in Oxford for about two months and then I started at Florence Treloar School in Hampshire. The boys' and girls' schools, Lord Mayor Treloar and Florence Treloar schools, were later amalgamated. It was all quite a wrench, because our family lived in Lincoln, and over the space of a year I was in hospital for six months, home for three months and then away again. I didn't get on very well at boarding school because the regime was very strict, but apart from that I think it was too much, going straight from hospital to boarding school. I did meet some lovely people there, though, who are still my friends today, although I only stayed there a year.

I left because I just couldn't settle, I don't really know why. I went from there to a college in Coventry, Hereward Education College, when I was fifteen. They were brand new, just opened, and they started with six students. They took me a year early, basically, I suppose, because they didn't have many students and I loved it there; it was so different from Treloar. I did four O levels and two A levels at college, and then I went from there to Sussex University, where I studied history.

I had some very good times at Sussex, and some bad times. My health suffered there, and I can understand why in hindsight, because it was the first time they'd provided accommodation for severely disabled students. They didn't provide twenty-four hour care, they only provided it from eight o'clock at night until ten in the morning. Now I would say that that was too little, but it was quite a challenge. I wanted to be there and I wanted to do it, so I just went on and did it. I did have some bad periods of being ill there, but I came out with a degree.

I had to have a year off in the middle because I became very poorly but that in its own way gave me more experience. I was allowed a year off but after being in hospital for six months, I went straight back to the university. Although I wasn't studying, I got elected on to the students' union, and I also did some work experience in Brighton Library and at a local school as a teacher's assistant, so I did quite a lot. Then I went back, did my final year and got my honours degree, a II:ii.

I was called chairperson of welfare for the students' union. I prepared information and factsheets on facilities and such like. I suppose I was beginning to realize that there were issues concerning disability that needed addressing, but everybody was too naive to know how to set about it. There were a couple of other students with disabilities where I was in the accommodation block, and we used to have quite in-depth discussions about issues, but we never actually did anything about it.

We'd talk about the problems of access round the campus and the difficulties of getting to lectures, about being aware that we were treated slightly differently. We were just generally, slowly, becoming aware that we weren't quite the same as other people, without quite being able to put our fingers on it. We wanted to challenge this attitude, but again we didn't really know how to.

I lived, with four other disabled students, in a special bungalow-type block called Kulukundis House, funded by Elias Kulukundis. There were other disabled students on campus, but they were people who could basically care for their own needs. My friend Brenda Robbins and I used to have these long discussions on disability. It's quite interesting because she lives in London and went on to become quite involved with the politics of disability, so I suppose you could say it was a breeding ground for people to start examining the things that we'd talked about.

When I finished university it was as if there really wasn't anywhere else to go. A social worker used to come to see us at Sussex. I'm not really quite sure why the university felt the need for these sort of people, but anyway when it actually came down to requesting help about what to do next – i.e. to get accommodation with support – he didn't have any ideas whatsoever. Neither did the careers adviser. Another able-bodied student I knew wanted to do social work, as I did, so when she got application forms for herself she got them for me as well. She was an economics student and had done nothing to do with social issues at all, while I had done quite a bit and had been on the student union. I didn't get one interview while she got interviews from everybody to do a CQSW in social work. That made me feel that basically all was not fair out there. The only interview I got was a pre-interview with Derbyshire Social Service. The man who interviewed me said he could not consider training me as a social worker, but if I wanted to work for the social services department in some capacity or other, they might consider it: he said he had seen disabled people get into the lift in the morning, so he thought that they did employ disabled people.

So that was it, really. I ended up going from a quite exciting life at university back home to Mum and Dad, which was a bit of a blow. I learned to drive when I was at home. I bought a car and tried to get a job. I went for several interviews but didn't achieve anything. Those were the times when I really did feel that there was a lot of prejudice about, the way the interviews were taken, and it always ended up with them saying things like could I make the tea and wanting to know if I could use a kettle.

I decided then that there wasn't a lot of point worrying too much about getting a job until I'd decided where I wanted to live. I didn't want to live at home with my Mum and Dad, I wanted a place of my own. That became my next challenge. I nearly got a flat near to where my parents lived, but for various reasons, like alterations it needed, that fell through. Then I got offered a flat at a place called Grove Road in Sutton-in-Ashfield, between Nottingham and Mansfield, which is quite a well-known accommodation place now. It was started by a couple of tetraplegics, a man and wife, who wanted to move out of Stoke Mandeville. They approached a housing association to build accommodation where severely disabled people might live, and there are three flats downstairs for disabled people and three flats upstairs for helpers. They had a flat free, so I scrubbed the idea of living near my Mum and Dad – well, it's not that far away – and went to live there, and was there for eleven years. While I lived there I did learn to be independent. I learned to drive and I did various kinds of voluntary work. I used to work in the CVS, the Council for Voluntary Service. I was their volunteer co-ordinator. People would come in wanting to do voluntary work, and I had to find them placements. I also got involved on the periphery of disability issues, because Ken and Maggie Davies, who then lived at Grove Road, were the first people to start the disability movement. I was involved with DIAL (Disability Information and Advice Line) and various things like that, and I was also very involved with sport. I think sport was wonderful really, because all through the summer there were loads of competitions to go to and we just had really good fun. I got in to the British teams for swimming, table tennis and fencing, so I used to do a lot of training. I was never particularly bored or anything, as I always had plenty to do. Then I was ill for about two years and was in hospital for that time. When I came out it was like being newly disabled all over again because I was nowhere near as fit as I had been before and I had to really make my life again. I couldn't just go back to where I'd been so I did an MA in women's studies at Sheffield Polytechnic, as well as various computer courses, got a part-time job at Nottingham University with the careers guidance people – and just got my travel expenses and did data input – then I got a job with Derbyshire Centre for Integrated Living as a community worker. Then I went on a holiday to Israel, met Mike, and that's it, I moved here. That was five years ago. I got a job with Cambridge City Council which enabled us to get the mortgage, so that's my potted history.

I think I've got a very stubborn streak so, although I don't think I'm a particularly forceful person, equally I'm not easily pushed aside. I don't think I'm either an optimist or a pessimist, although I do always think about the negative aspects of things. Whenever I do try to do something, I always think of what could go wrong, but that wouldn't actually prevent me from doing it. I have had times when I've been very depressed, but I don't think it lasts for an awfully long time, basically because I get bored with myself. I suppose when I think of people whose company I enjoy, they are people who do and talk about interesting things, even if it's just what films they've watched or what books they've read. I don't necessarily mean people who've travelled the world, it's just people who've got interesting minds, so that even if I've not felt able to go out and about, I've always tried to keep myself interested and interesting.

There have only been three main times when I've felt depressed, and each time it was because I felt trapped. The first time was at that special school. It's not having a choice: you're there, and as far as everyone's concerned you're going to be there for good, even though that might not be what you want. When I left university, I felt trapped at home, and I was very depressed in hospital, because for a long period of time nobody knew how to get me better. As long as I feel that I've got a way out of things, then I don't get depressed.

I am aware, particularly now that I work in a completely able-bodied world, that I have a significantly different view of life to that of any of my colleagues. When you meet another disabled person, you do have a common ground that you don't have with able-bodied people; that doesn't mean that you'll get on with them any better, but there is certainly a link, a common experience. But I can't look at myself objectively and see why I feel so different to my colleagues at work. I just know that sometimes I talk about things and I know they haven't got a clue what I'm talking about.

I haven't ever really thought about what my life would have been like if I wasn't disabled. I remember at university I used to have a lecturer who was very interested in what I thought about things, and what I wanted to do when I left university. His way of trying to look at what I could do when I left was to try and find out what I thought I would have done had I not become disabled. At the end of the day, it wasn't very helpful.

I don't think my life's ever been boring. The side of disability that is the downer is the medical problems that you have no control over. If all that being disabled was about was not being able to walk and being in a wheelchair, then that would not have been a problem: it's low energy levels, infections and stuff like that that present difficulties. But you've just got to get on with it.

The biggest influence in your life when you're first disabled is the doctor, the specialist. I remember my specialist finding out that I was going to university, and he told me I was absolutely mad, and that what I should be doing was staying at home with my Mum – you know, just accepting that that was where my life was going to be. So actually to get to university and, despite the health problems, get a degree the same as anybody else, was quite an achievement. Another achievement was when I moved into a flat on my own, because in those days these things weren't the norm. Somebody said to me that I'd never do it, therefore I had to go and do it.

Then I started to do sport. Sport has always been, and to some extent will always be, an area for very fit paraplegic men and women, and tetraplegics with my level of injury are not usually in the forefront. You have to know what you're looking at to know whether I'm a good fencer or not, but I was very fortunate to have Les Veal as a fencing coach. He was trying to raise the profile of fencing for very severely disabled people, and he picked me to go to what they called the Internationals. It sent quite a few shock-waves through the establishment because that meant the organizers had to provide more care support; usually the people who went on these things were very independent and didn't need any care. Again, I found that quite good. I didn't ever win a gold medal for anything, but I think I got the silver a few times. I suppose I do get pleasure out of challenging people's assumptions, so that was also good. I do a lot of swimming as well, which I'm sure toughens you up. I had a lot of problems with my leg, and was in hospital for a couple of years. When I came out it took a lot of fighting to get back to doing something that I wanted to do. Again there were those assumptions that I wouldn't do anything else, that I would just stay and be looked after. I do need care input, but I also want to be able to do things for myself. I still feel shocked sometimes by what medical people can say to you, and I find myself wondering where on earth they get their ideas from. I was at the spinal unit a few weeks ago and one of the specialists happened to see me as I went out the door. 'I hear you're working part-time,' he said, and I said, 'Full-time actually.' He went on, 'That's always been your problem, wanting too much out of life!' He hadn't seen me for ten years and yet he could make a bold statement like that. When you imagine how some disabled people actually rely on a specialist to give them confidence to go out and do things. . . . People like that specialist have got a blinkered view of disabled people, and think that it's completely out of order that you do what you feel able to do. I wouldn't do it if I didn't feel that I was able to do it. There may come a time when I'm not able to work full-time, but I can at the moment, and that's my decision. Being able to work, take part in sports and live independently is my greatest achievement.

I think I've been very lucky in the sense that disablement does enable you to meet some really nice people that you perhaps wouldn't meet otherwise. It also makes you look at areas open to you, that perhaps you wouldn't necessarily have thought of, like fencing. I mean, the only reason

I started to fence was because Les saw me one day at the sports centre, and said, 'Have a go.' When opportunities arose, I went for them when perhaps I wouldn't have done otherwise, and I have met some really nice people. I have started carriage-driving (with a horse and carriage) since I lived down here. That's opened up a world of people that I wouldn't normally have come into contact with.

Sadly, since I've been working I've not done a lot of exercise and it's something that I'm very conscious of. I know that I'm not as fit as when I lived up in Sutton-in-Ashfield. There was the sports club at the hospital and the local sports centre that was geared to allowing you to go swimming. I did swim once or twice a week and I went to fitness to do a bit of weight training. I do miss it, but there isn't the disability awareness around here, and Haverhill swimming pool hasn't got an accessible changing room at the moment. I know that if I were really disciplined and could get my act together, I really ought to do it. Mike and I went on holiday to Israel just before Christmas, and we both realized that we were both unfit. He's now trying to get back into being fit again, and it's one of the things that I will do, but tomorrow.

I haven't found, in general, that people in sport have preconceptions about disability that need to be overcome, though sometimes the judges need a word or two in their ears to make them understand. There's a long way to go, I think, but because of having been so ill and therefore having become more disabled than I was, I thought that my opportunities for doing risky things were probably gone. It isn't exactly risky, carriage-driving, but there is always an element of risk with horses. To be able to go off across fields in the country has been really nice, because I'm not able to do it normally.

Disability has given me many problems to tackle and overcome. The first one was that specialist at Lodge Moor, but we're talking about a long time ago, and things have changed quite a bit since. There was an expectation then that women who were disabled didn't get the same rehabilitation as men; there was a lower expectation of what they would achieve. It was assumed that you would go home and spend the rest of your life with your parents, and indeed many people did. If that's what they want, that's fine, but I wanted to do a bit more than that. I think there's a lot of discrimination by the medical profession – low expectations of what you can do, and an assumption that you are going to do what they say. I always find it quite amazing that people who don't know you from Adam can assume that they have the right to tell you what you can and can't do. An example of this attitude was that doctor saying that I was mad to be going to university, although I know that in later years, he thought a lot of me, and was quite proud of what I'd done. There is this attitude from the medical profession that you need to be kept in cottonwool almost, and I can understand where they're coming from, but it's not real life.

I think I've always found the worst discrimination on a wider scale is in employment and housing. I always feel I can cope to a certain extent when I go to a restaurant and find that I can't get into it – so you fight for better access, or you find somewhere else to go. But when people actually stop you from doing something and that affects the whole of your life – if you can't get work – then that totally restricts your whole life's opportunities. Those are the things that I find the most difficult. Trying to find somewhere to live, for instance. If you can't get into one restaurant, you can get into another, but if you can't find somewhere to live, you're talking about having to move, say, to the other side of the country. Mike and I had to wait three years before we could live together, because we couldn't find anywhere suitable.

Mike worked down here in Haverhill, and I worked up in Derbyshire, and after a year or eighteen months we wanted to live together. Initially, I don't think we worried too much about me working, we thought we'd just move in together, and I'd get some work if I could, but that just wasn't an option. The sort of properties you need have to be very spacious to accommodate a wheelchair, so we couldn't afford anywhere. The council hadn't got anywhere, and that was it. That put a strain on the relationship. Then Mike decided that he would try and move up north because I did have a flat there, but he couldn't get a job up north, and was feeling really depressed about the whole thing. The other thing was actually trying to find a house that we could afford and we could adapt. Social services in Derbyshire were being very unpleasant. I worked for Derbyshire Centre for Integrated Living and they were making it very clear that my working for them didn't mean that I could get preferential treatment. Then I saw an advert in the *Guardian* for this job in Cambridge. We were going on holiday down here anyway, and I got the application form the morning we were leaving, so I filled it in when I was on holiday. I got the job, and that gave us enough buying power to get a mortgage on this bungalow. This is the only place in two or three years of looking that we could actually have thought of living in for the six months it took to adapt it properly. People think that when you go out to buy a property or to move into a property that you're going to have choice, but that just isn't true. If you haven't got any money – like compensation – you really don't have much choice. We didn't have any problems with getting the house adapted, but we did have to move in before it was done because I needed to start work as soon as possible. We might want to think about moving again, but the practicalities are also very discriminatory, because, as I said, there just aren't the premises that are accessible to move into.

I had encountered the same lack of choice when I was looking for a job. I suppose for a long time I gave up looking because I just kept getting so many refusals. That's why I went into sport. The only real reason I actually took up employment was because, after being ill, I was in touch with a friend who's also disabled, Elizabeth Standon. She used to work at Nottingham University doing a project on disabled graduates – where are they now, sort of thing – and she wrote to me with a huge questionnaire. I wrote back very curtly because I didn't think there was any point filling it in – you know, I'd had zilch opportunities, and it was all a waste of time. Anyway she always said afterwards that my letter had really upset her. Eventually she enabled me to go and start doing the data inputting for their project, and they worked very hard to give me the confidence to start looking for work again. More jobs were becoming available then that were specifically targeted for disabled people, so there was more opportunity than when I had first started to look. That was my first major failure, after university, not being able to get employment or interviews for anything.

There are other things that I often think about doing and there are lots of times when I think about going for other jobs or doing other courses, but I'm slightly held back by a lack of energy and being a bit fearful. I have a good job now and I'm a bit frightened of trying anything new for fear of not being able to actually do it. I'm not really sure how much further I can push myself.

Mike is very good at assuming I will be able to manage, and that gives me confidence. If I can't do whatever he wants to do – like riding or whatever – I do my best to make sure that he doesn't feel that I'm holding him back. Equally he's quite happy with what we do, but when he does need to go away for a few days for work reasons and that sort of thing, he appears never to assume that I won't be able to manage. That's quite nice because I never feel that I've got somebody who's worried about me. I mean, he will worry, obviously, but not to an overpowering extent.

I think my disability must have been very hard for my parents to come to terms with, primarily because of the way disability was handled in those days. It wasn't done well. I mean, you have your accident and that's it. My parents lived in Lincoln, and I was in hospital in Sheffield, so we were immediately wrenched apart. Nowadays in Lodge Moor, there's no limit on visiting hours, but when I had my accident I was only allowed visitors on Wednesdays, Saturdays and Sundays, between set hours. When visiting time was finished that was it. Neither was there any counselling, no sort of discussion about emotional things at all; it was a case of this is how it is, very matter-of-fact. When your time in hospital had finished you went home, and there was no gradual process of building up to it and getting used to things: on a particular date you were just discharged. My parents' house was not adapted, it was an ordinary detached three-bedroomed house, so I moved into the living room. We had a tin bath in the kitchen, and that was it. Then I got told I was being sent away to school and that was it again.

Dad's job on the railway in Lincoln closed, and he got moved to Sheffield where they bought a bungalow, so when I went home on holiday I was able to stay with them in better circumstances. I'm lucky in the sense that I come from a family which is very practical; there's all sorts of traumas going on, but we just deal with the here and now. I think that's probably been very helpful, you just have to get on with it.

One of the saddest things of all was that I lost all my friends after my accident. First I was in hospital, then I went to a new school, then we moved house and that was it. That's really where sport was a lifeline, because it enabled me to meet people of my own age.

In an ideal world I'd love a slightly bigger house. My house is lovely, and I love everything about it, but it's just a little bit on the small side for getting in at the doors and around, and you're limited to what wheelchair you can use. I would really like a detached property which is slightly bigger, with an integrated bathroom within my own bedroom so I wouldn't have to come out into the corridor. I don't know what the likelihood of that is because a) such a house has got to become available and b) we've got to be able to afford it.

I've certainly thought about having children, I've just never fallen pregnant. It's just not something that happened. I think a lot about ageing now, too. I read a book recently about ageing with disability, and it is something I'm conscious of. I'm sure it's true that you don't have as much energy as you did, but then I do work full-time and I have done only for the last six or seven years. Working full-time is incredibly tiring, so which comes first I don't know really. Having had that bout of illness a few years ago, I know that my health's not as good as it used to be. I am conscious anyway that disability is not static, and that you have to be aware of things changing.

When I went to work for the Derbyshire Centre for Integrated Living I think that gave me an enormous opportunity. To be paid for something and to realize you've got skills that people actually value, is an enormous lift to your self-esteem and confidence. I don't think that can ever be underestimated. I worked for them for two and a half years and I would have continued to work for them had I not had to move down here. Working for Cambridge City Council has also been quite an eye-opener because of being in an all able-bodied environment. In many respects Cambridge City Council are very good, and they have tried to be accommodating, but equally I try not to draw attention to myself, although in many respects I can't help it.

My job was to set up a taxi card scheme and a shop mobility scheme to start off with. But I'm not somebody who can sit around not doing an awful lot, and I did have spare capacity, so I was taken on two days a week to work in our policy department to look at disability policy throughout the Council. I have done quite a lot of work on access and just generally raising the profile of consultation with disabled people, but one thing I have found, and which I'm trying to challenge at the moment, is that anything to do with disability comes automatically to me. I'm doing three jobs in one job's time, and I'm finding it a bit of a strain at the moment. Very unusually, I have lost my temper a couple of times recently, and I think people are suddenly realizing that perhaps there is a problem simply because I'm so tired, because I'm not given any support. I have requested that this is addressed.

Sometimes when I am very tired, I wonder why I'm doing all this work. It hits me particularly in the winter time because we have to get up at six o'clock in the morning. Mike's work starts at a quarter to eight, I have to get into Cambridge, and it's twenty-seven miles at peak-time traffic, and takes up to an hour and a quarter to get there. When it's cold and snowing, and nobody in their right minds would go out, I've got to turn out and it's then that I really wish I had the time and support to investigate other things that I could do. It would be good to do more from home, but that isn't something I've got the opportunity to do at the moment. Maybe one day I will, but the fact is that I have got skills within the disability area that are actually required at the moment, and I'm quite happy to be paid for that. When the time comes, and it probably will come, when there is nothing left for me to do, then I'll have to think seriously about whether I'm just paid for being a disabled person. I'm sure they'll recognize that as well, but it isn't a problem at the moment, so I'm quite happy to be employed for the skills that I have. I'm not knocking it, because it has enabled me to work.

I'm not worried about being pigeonholed at the moment because that was the job I wanted, and as I say, it gives me an opportunity to look at how disability is addressed across the Council, and I think I have done quite a bit.

I don't particularly like the job title I've got now. It was Disabled Person's Transport Co-ordinator, but now it's Special Needs Policy Officer. Although I don't like the title Special Needs, the reason they chose that was because it meant that I was available to do work on a lot of varying issues. It need not necessarily be disability, it could be other areas. I suppose you could argue that 'special needs' includes anything within equal opportunities. However, they didn't want to go down that equal-opportunities avenue, because they are trying to get all departments to take equal opportunities on board. They didn't want to label me in that way as a result.

The medical profession is one of the areas that I find most difficult. They have so much power over you, and they're very difficult to challenge because they are the holders of the information. You've got to be incredibly strong to challenge them, and if you're not feeling very well, that's an awful burden to put on yourself. Basically, you've got to find somebody that you trust and once you've found that person you've got to go with them. I know, because when I was ill, some people used to say, 'Well, I don't know why you don't get a second opinion, we've always had second and third opinions.' Well, that's fine, but you've got to have energy to do that, and at the end of the day, if you trust your doctors you have to trust their judgement and, rightly or wrongly, have got to go with it in the end. I am lucky in that I have a consultant whom I trust. It does worry me, in that I've had one consultant retire, and I was lucky to trust the next one. I'd be very worried if I outlive his retirement. It's just that the medical profession are very difficult to deal with.

My experience of hospital in general was a mixture of good and bad. What it's like being in hospital depends on who's in at the same time. I found that, when I had my two-year spell in, if you've got really good people that are either funny or interesting, time goes by very quickly. If you've got a lot of people who are a lot older than you, it's not so good. When I had my accident I was thirteen and for a long time I was the only child surrounded by grown men. Then a couple of young girls with spina bifida came in for sore repairs; they were sixteen, and the hospital moved us three into a side ward and that was quite fun. But of course they moved on, and it was back to being with the blokes again. There were a couple of times when people came in who had mental health problem; were injured as a result of suicide attempts, and that was a bit unpleasant for somebody very young like me.

I find it really depressing that they will close Lodge Moor at the end of 1994. It was an old building, but it was out on the moors and it was really lovely. You looked out of your window at all the fields. It's being closed down, sold off, and the spinal unit is now going to be in a hospital in the centre of Sheffield.

I believe that alternative and conventional medicine complement one another. I'm not someone who's ever thought that if I went down the herbalist path, I'd stop everything else. I have taken herbal stuff, and had acupuncture and reflexology and all those sort of things, and I have found them very beneficial. I think they can help raise your physical well-being generally. I still go for periods of reflexology, particularly in winter, I use oils and things, and I'm always reading books on alternative food.

I'm sure that it is just common sense to eat a lot of very good food, raw vegetables and all that sort of thing. Massages and things like that should help your circulation and anything to help you relax should be good. They might not cure, but they certainly help you to cope. I think reflexology and massage are the best ones for me, because I find them very relaxing.

The problem with medical research into spinal injury is that it always seems to set its sights on getting people walking again. Obviously that is incredibly important for new injuries, but I don't see it as something that's going to help me in my particular circumstances. Yes, I hope that they are successful, but there must be research going on into infection control and things like that. I'd be more interested in hearing about research into long-term chronic complaints, but somehow I never pick up on that. I'd be happier if there was more concentration on the more practical, less dramatic details of living with spinal injury.

When I came home from hospital, I wasn't rehabilitated really. It was only when I went to Oxford, to Mary Marlborough Lodge, that I learned anything. Young physios from Stoke Mandeville did a lot of very practical sort of stuff, transferring me and getting me in and out of cars, which was, I suppose, one of the first inklings I had that you could actually have quite a normal life. I think it's very difficult to achieve that in hospital.

When I got my job in Cambridge, one of the provisos they made about me having the job was that I shouldn't need any help from any member of staff. I said, 'Well, the only help I need is to get in and out of the car'. They weren't very happy about that, but I said that I would investigate what other alternatives were on the market, hoists and things. The bottom line was that there isn't anything suitable apart from transit vans. So I've leased a transit van from the Council, and I've got grants towards the alterations. I've now got this electric wheelchair, so life's a lot easier. That's another tie to work, really, as I'm not sure that I can afford a van. It's a vicious circle, but that's the sort of transport where you don't need to get out of your chair to drive. Before I was ill, at a push I could get in and out of the car myself, but afterwards that was it, really – it did put the mockers on independence completely.

I also use the train and quite enjoy it. I wish buses were accessible – it would make life a lot easier if they were – and I use taxis. I do use the public transport that is available, and I think it's wrong that more isn't.

I once heard somebody say that when you are disabled, you lose your spontaneity, and that is true: you've got to have the energy and that's something that's sadly lacking. If everything were adapted to your needs – your ramp here and your hoist there, your van here and the electric wheelchair there – that would be really good. But you have to be conscious that as soon as you go outside your front door, the world out there is not like that, and that's a problem.

I think you've got to try and find out as much information about things as you can. Now, whenever I go anywhere, I always make sure that I've contacted local disability organizations to find out which hotels have the best access and so on, so that I can make a choice, and make it on sound ground. I also think because I am a stubborn person, whatever I've really wanted I've worked towards. Why shouldn't I go to college and university, for instance? They should be accessible to disabled people, and therefore if you have the ability to reach that level of education, you should go for it. There are places around that can enable you to do it. It's the same with living independently: why shouldn't I live that way? Finding other disabled people who'd already done it was important to me, finding people who echoed my own beliefs. Living independently is an option for everybody at various levels, and you shouldn't be put off either by able-bodied people or by professional people who say, 'Oh I wouldn't do that.' Although it's taken a long time to find employment, again it's going against the view that disabled people can't work, again it's finding the right thing for you, how many hours you can do, and keeping on trying to do it. Once more it's finding other disabled people who've done it, and finding the support to enable you to do it. I've always found that possibly my biggest support is other disabled people's experiences, and their faith that disabled people can do it. I found it very disappointing when I moved down here to Suffolk and indeed Cambridge, and found that there weren't many disabled groups. There are more now, but when I was in Derbyshire and Yorkshire there were many very strong disabled groups, whether sports groups or political groups. To come down here, and find there was nothing, was really awful. As a result, there aren't as many accessible places here. I'd taken a lot of things for granted because the disability movement had already moved various things forward further north; they're only slowly being moved down here.

People are at their least helpful when they think they're helping you, but are acting without consulting you, so they're making an assumption about what you need. If you then say, 'But that's not what I want done,' you get a backlash almost, because they feel hurt. Because they think they're doing something to help you, they're sort of shocked because they feel you've rebuffed them. If a complete stranger says to me when I have my car, 'Do you need a hand?,' I don't feel guilty about saying 'No, thank you' or 'Yes, please', depending on whether it's appropriate, but I sometimes find it difficult to say no to people I see regularly. They're the ones that are most difficult because they think they know you and what you need. I know that it is their problem, but when you point out that they don't know, it's quite difficult when it comes to seeing them again and you've made a stand about it.

It depends on the person really. I'm probably my own worst enemy in some respects because I tend to let things go for quite a long time when I know that people are only trying to be helpful. It's when you get tired and somebody does something that you suddenly think 'Not again!' and you tackle them. It's like a bolt out of the blue to them, and you realize that you should have warned them before that it wasn't appropriate. In certain circumstances, when I've calmed down, I've always gone back to people and said 'Look, the reason I lost my temper was . . .' or 'The reason I said that was because you didn't ask me first, you made an assumption.' They've said, 'Well, I know you can't do this, so I thought I'd do that,' and I say, 'Well, how do you know I can't do that, you never asked me.' You can see that they haven't really thought about that, so that's hard. It's not always the easiest thing, going back to people to talk it through, but I do try. That is the main problem with well-meaning people.

I can't say my disability's never got me down because, as I've said, there have been times when I've felt very trapped and very low. I think all in all, though, that I've come out of it reasonably well. I am stubborn, I do get cross, and I do get on my soapbox sometimes about things, but I don't feel that I'm particularly bitter about it because I don't see it in that way. Equally I don't think I can say that everything's wonderful, because of health problems which I wish I didn't have. It's not the not walking, I mean I've never had that sort of long-term worry about not walking. If I had 100 percent energy levels and never had to worry about having an infection, then I could say that, on the whole I'm reasonably well balanced. Sometimes I wish I could do this, that or the other, but then Mike says that as well, that there are loads of things he wishes he could do. But that's life really, isn't it?

I hate it when people say, 'Oh, I think you're marvellous, I don't know how you manage to get to work five days a week.' I'll say, 'Well, I'll tell you how, I'm absolutely knackered on Fridays!' I find it quite difficult that people think, because you appear on the surface to lead a 'normal life', that you're somehow a bit odd. I always want to put people down a bit when they say that. They seem really surprised when I do things, because when an able-bodied person looks at a disabled person, they try to see themselves under those circumstances and they just can't do it. They don't seem to see that life does go on, and that we cope very well, thank you.

As far as up until I started work, I'd had absolutely no money, so I got all the available benefits without any trouble. The problem came when I started to work because, as far as the benefits system is concerned, if you're disabled you don't work, and if you work you're not disabled. Because I had all my disability benefits stopped, I had to get an MP involved. There was just this view from the social security side that, because I was only working part-time, I was still entitled to certain of my disability benefits. The bureaucratic side held to a hard and fast rule, and therefore I must be lying if I said I was working and disabled, because that is their definition of disability, being unable to work.

If I had a free hand, I'd say that disabled people need an overall level of disability benefit. I feel very vulnerable now because I worry about a drop in my standard of living if I had to give up work. I find that an unwelcome and unnecessary additional pressure. I think if you have to give up work because you're not fit enough, you should feel that you are going to get various benefits and support, but that isn't the case, or at least I don't believe it is.

I would like to see an anti-discrimination law. Because I work in a local authority, I can see that things definitely move on disability when it's a requirement by law – the building control officers ensure new buildings are accessible, for instance. As soon as you start talking to architects working outside the public sector, though, it's purely dependent on the individual that you get. Certain things have come in through the Citizens' Charter, and local government has to meet various standards: everybody has to say which of their public buildings are accessible and which aren't, and what they are going to do about it if they're not. I can see that when you have to do something, you take it on board, but if you don't have to do it, because you've got so many other things you have to do, that one thing becomes a lower priority. It always seems to me that people think that they're doing the disabled a favour, but it shouldn't be like that: you shouldn't be getting access because they're doing you a favour, they should be doing it because they've got to, because it's part of building regulations. It's your right to have it; you should have things as a right, and you haven't.

Because I'm having to confront people's prejudices all the time at work, I can quite easily see how difficult it is sometimes for people. Sometimes when I come home and I find there's a letter saying, 'Please write to your local MP about such and such', I think that I can't do that, that I just haven't got the energy or the time to do it. I don't want to live my life twenty-four hours a day to promote access for the disabled, but I do try to be as visible as possible. If something isn't accessible, then I like to make a point of making people aware of it, but equally, if somebody does do something and they've made really good provision, then I try to find the person who has been responsible to say thank you, so that they know it has been worthwhile.

I think legislation is vital in promoting disability awareness. It's all right if you work in a field where disability has a high profile, because there you're going to get a high level of awareness, but disabled people shouldn't just be channelled into certain areas, they should have open access to everything. Unless there's legislation, however, you can't achieve that, because if a person can say, 'Well, no disabled people come into my building', no amount of awareness-raising is going to get them to change it. It's like transport: unless there are regulations to make companies buy low-floored buses, how on earth are they going to be forced to make the amount of expenditure required, I can't see them doing it voluntarily.

I try to make sure we do go on holiday, as I do like to travel. I'm a bit nervous of going too far away, as I'm not sure how good my health will be. One day, I may get as far as Canada. I like mountains and I've heard good reports about it as far as disability goes. I admire disabled people who've been to India and places like that, and I know that there are organizations to help disabled people do those sort of things. There are a lot more opportunities for younger disabled people to do adventurous things, but I think – not just because I'm older but because I just have a different feeling about holidays now – that I want to go away and be relaxed. I'm a bit more geared to wanting nicer hotels. I like going to Italy, I think that's a lovely country, and I like the people. I also like France. The furthest I've been is Israel, which I like very much. Mike would like to do more adventurous things, but whether we will, I don't know.

Going to Israel was quite daring. I didn't tell my specialist that I was going because it was after I'd been very ill, but I just felt that I had to do something to break the way my life was going. So I went with a holiday group that organizes tours for disabled people and people were a bit amazed. I didn't actually tell many people I was going because I didn't want them exclaiming before I went and saying 'I told you so' if anything went wrong. It was quite an adventure, the first time I'd ever been outside Europe. That was good – I do think that people should have a challenge. I think I said earlier that it's up to the individual what challenges they need to take on, but I'm the sort of person who needs to set challenges for myself, otherwise I get this feeling of not achieving anything.

Before going on holiday, I ring up the Spinal Injury Association and get guidance as to what places are like, because there's nothing worse than not having an accessible bathroom, for instance. When you go away you want to enjoy yourself, you don't want to have to suffer, so I always try to make sure that I'm armed with good information and I have been very lucky. Before I met Mike I used organizations like ACROSS and the Phoenix Trust to help me go on holiday, simply because my parents are getting older. I'm lucky in that my sister used to take me abroad when she could but it was nice to go away with groups of people and be a bit adventurous, but at the same time feeling reasonably safe because I'd got care on hand. I'm always looking for the next holiday!

The single most important piece of advice I'd give to anyone who's sustained a spinal injury is: Give yourself time. I know that for the first year, probably more, everything seems daunting. It does take time for your body to adjust, and there will always be those people who are more capable than you, but you shouldn't let that put you off. Everybody can achieve anything they want, given their own time and pace. You should look for opportunities: somebody once said to me, 'What's for you won't go by you, but it won't come to you without you doing the groundwork.' Just because you apply for one job, and don't get it, doesn't mean to say that nobody will have you, but if you don't keep applying then nobody's going to know you're there. I suppose that's one of the things that I believe: whenever it's ready for me, whatever I want to do next will happen if it was meant to.

Tim Marshall

Tim Marshall was born in 1946 and works as a senior lecturer in public health and epidemiology at Birmingham University Medical School. He is married, and sustained his spinal injury in 1972 in a climbing accident.

I'd driven up with a friend from Birmingham to Derbyshire on a Saturday morning in September 1972 to go climbing on the Gritstone Edges. We went up and down and up and down, which you do there as they are mostly single-pitch climbs. Towards the end of the day I was leading on some route or other, and, too far above my running belay for that to be of any use in the event of an accident, I got off balance. I tried to pull up on finger jams, but blood ran out, and I just fell off, down about twenty feet, landing full square on the ground which gave me a compression fracture. After I landed, apparently I tipped over backwards and bounced around a few rocks, but my crash helmet saved my life. I was then taken to Chesterfield Royal Infirmary on the Saturday evening, and on the Monday up to the spinal unit at Sheffield where I stayed for the next eight months. I was briefly, maybe a couple of minutes, knocked out after landing, and I knew as soon as I came round that I couldn't feel my legs. I didn't know then that sometimes you can get what's known as spinal shock and you can recover from it, but I never assumed any such thing. As soon as I realized I couldn't feel my legs, I thought, oh shit, here we go. As it happened, I didn't get any feeling back.

My break was T9 complete, and after I was operated on for a spinal cyst which developed later, in 1988, I went up to about T6 – if you can have such a thing – that's in terms of anatomical level. What happens in the operation is they snap the back off the vertebrae and chop into the spinal cord to let the cyst whoosh itself out. When people have gallstones or kidney stones, they often end up in a bottle on their desks. I wanted a bit of spinal cord as not many people have their own spinal cord on their desk! My wife says that it's revolting and disgusting, but unfortunately they took it all away to do some histology on so I never got hold of any. I suspect that would be very nearly a first, very few people can have their own spinal cord in a bottle in front of them. I didn't manage it, I'm sorry to say.

There was little active treatment in those days in the acute stages of management of spinal injury. Nowadays they pile in anti-coagulants to stop people having bloodclots, but that hadn't begun when I was injured. I was conscious enough on the Saturday evening to give names, addresses and telephone numbers of people to contact. So the first visitor was my Mum who came up on the Sunday morning, and the next visitors I think were on Tuesday in the spinal unit. So that was pretty quick. The social support I had from friends while I was in hospital was superb. Sheffield was located more or less midway between Nottingham, Birmingham, Manchester and Leeds where I had friends or relatives, so people piled in to see me. That was good, I enjoyed that, and found it very supportive.

So far as the management of the injury was concerned it was fairly conventional. It was a compression fracture, superficially not very severe as judged from the x-rays, but still the landing had done its damage. I was kept in the acute ward for rather longer than people would be nowadays because I couldn't pee, and the bladder management took a long time to get going. It was interesting in that it was like growing up again in a very compressed period: in the acute ward all the staff were female and to start with you were mothered and everything was done for you; then, at an appropriate time, for the men anyway, you were sent off down to the men's rehab ward which was pretty rough and tough, where there were mixed staff, and you learned to grow up. It was a very masculine environment, partly, I guess, because of the kind of people who were at that time the predominant source of spinal injury – there were men with industrial injuries, younger ones with motor-bike injuries, and silly ones like me with sporting injuries. It was a much harsher and harder environment, just because of those people, and I didn't find that bit of the stay terribly comfortable because I wasn't part of a brash, male-dominated, male-orientated society. My social circle wasn't like that.

Overall, insofar as you can enjoy such things, I enjoyed the stay in hospital. The two people I got on best with were my physio, who was a male remedial gymnast (it was he who introduced me to the sport side of things), and the sister on the acute ward. She was a superb nurse and she could beat me at Scrabble which put her a long way up in my estimation.

Physically and psychologically, I think my stay in hospital was very good. It was good for me then both in terms of what I was encouraged to do physically and, I think, psychologically certainly because of the relationship that developed with the physio and the sister in the acute ward. From a longer perspective looking back, I think there were some gross deficiencies in the place. If you weren't interested in sport or physical activity, for instance, nothing else was offered, there was nothing available and you were on your tod. There was a film show once a week, which was fine, but that wasn't an active participation. There's an awful lot of time during the day when, once you've started getting up, there is scope for all sorts of things to be offered to people, particularly in the evenings because you don't have to be in bed by seven o'clock.

From the point of view of getting advice on jobs, I'm not a good person to talk to because I knew my job was being kept open, I was very lucky. I did see people from the employment service coming in and talking to people, with what degree of success I don't know, but I would have thought that sort of advice is needed by every disabled person of working age. Again nothing was done about driving, and because of problems that the unit had had about people either escaping for an evening or running away or whatever, and coming back drunk, there was virtually an absolute ban on anybody going outside the hospital grounds. I think that was a mistake, but I don't think that's imposed as severely now, if it's imposed at all. People are encouraged to learn how to get out and about, and to discover what it feels like and how you can cope psychologically with being out there at four feet high instead of six feet high. I think that's very important, because discovering it for the first time when you are checked out, if that is the first time, can be a hell of a shock. It wasn't actually the first time for us because we had a fortnight out maybe a month before discharge to experience it. I think that's fine up to a point, but all you got when you went back was 'How did you get on then?' There was no psychological support in any formal sense, and I think there should be. You've got all sorts of fears, and the scope for articulating them is minimal unless you want to appear a complete fool amongst all the lads who were being brash and bold superficially, but were probably just as worried underneath. Again it's a male thing not to talk about how you feel, isn't it? Given the lack of any forum in which to do so, there's certainly no encouragement, and I think that's a shame.

When I left hospital in Sheffield I came home to my Mum's house to start with. She only had an upstairs loo, and so I used to have to bum my way up and down the stairs, up in the evening and down in the morning. That wasn't easy, and I'm not sure whether I could do it now.

The fact that my job had been held open was of enormous benefit, unquantifiable – I mean it's channelled the rest of my life since. My head of department kept my job open for me and without that I don't know what would have happened. Mum was then living in Evesham which is thirty-five miles away, and at that stage there was no sort of driving instruction while you were still an in-patient at a hospital. Going back to live with my Mum after I'd already broken the link wouldn't have been appropriate even if I had wanted to, but I couldn't go back to the house I'd been living in before the accident either. I wrote to the university accommodation office and people at work went to talk to them. Eventually somebody broke a log-jam of nothing happening by taking me off to a hall of residence, arranging to see the warden, and asking 'Could you put this guy up?' This was early July, and we found a way in which I could use one of the upstairs rooms. There was a tiny lift which an ordinary wheelchair wouldn't go into, but a small chair, the 8BL, could if you took one or possibly both hand rims off. Since it was only used to get into the room, that was fine, and basically I was put in there to start with because it was the summer vacation. I was put in an ordinary student room and I could actually use the loos. There weren't wheelchair loos, the place was in no sense designed for anybody in a wheelchair, but I found I could use them in this small chair. That's the most critical thing, if you've got a loo you can get to, then the rest more or less follows. But I couldn't stay there beyond the middle of September, because the students were coming back.

There was a box room which was used for student emergencies in late September and early October and they agreed to let me have it. I lived in this for a year, it was about five foot six by eleven feet! Then the university put some money towards building its first purpose-converted accommodation for disabled students. There'd been nothing up until then except an earlier conversion of the health centre, which had been done with an eye to disabled students living there. A new medical officer had come in and said, 'This is rubbish, the health centre is not the right place for a student to live.' So the university found some money from somewhere to put towards creating a couple of rooms. I had one of them, slightly bigger than the one I'd had before.

During my first year back, there was at least one, maybe two, vacant lectureships, and I was nudged into one of them. It's interesting, during the year before I fell, the department was re-writing courses. I wasn't brought in as a teaching person, though I'd done some, but they asked me to re-write the main epidemiology course for the third-year medical students, and so I spent most of my year doing this, and apparently it was a success. I didn't actually teach it the first year because I was in hospital, but, maybe on the strength of that work, they felt I was worth trying to hang on to. I think there was quite a bit of generosity on the university's part, or the department's part, because I certainly didn't have the kind of academic credentials which would normally have been regarded as grounds for giving somebody a lectureship.

Although I was registered for a PhD at that stage, I think it's fair to say that it ran into difficulties – I had disagreements with my supervisor and then he retired – and it just sort of fizzled out. It happens quite a lot.

I was given a lectureship and carried on teaching and developing courses. Getting a research programme together was a bit difficult in a sense because I didn't have a subject, although I had a methodology. In fact, what I did for quite a long time was advise clinicians: they would find their way to me and ask if I could advise them about how to design research, how to collect data, and how to analyse it. Sometimes I'd do it with them or occasionally for them, and sometimes I became a joint author, and so that goes on to the academic list of what you've done. In academic terms, I was asked to do some tutoring for some postgraduate people in 1975, and I actually developed what I think is probably the most successful of any of the programmes for tutoring people in what is now called public health medicine anywhere in the country: we had an overall pass rate in the region of 85 percent in the part one exam, while the national average at that time was about 65 to 70 percent. I know virtually all the consultants in public health medicine in the region because I've taught them all. I was promoted in about 1991 to senior lecturer and now, because of the changes that have occurred in the health authority at the regional level, my head of department has been seconded to the region, and I'm acting head of department at the moment which is causing some hassles, some pressures.

I've never had a life plan, I've never had a long-term perspective, most of the time I'm just looking two to three years ahead at what's coming on the horizon. I have tried applying for jobs elsewhere and never been successful. I was head-hunted the other month but didn't want the job. It was for a chair actually, but I think they were getting desperate, I'd better not say where...

At the professional level, what I'm particularly concerned with is getting good delivery and good teaching to the students, and, with luck, enthusing some of them. There is also the research side of things which we have to pay more attention to nowadays, and that's something of a concern, particularly in fairly recent years. It goes back to the fact that I don't have a major subject speciality, and the way you make your name in academic circles is to become the world's expert on something or other. I'm not that, and never will be.

In a sense, I'm interdisciplinary and that presents problems when external experts are reviewing the academic excellence of my work, I guess, because I'm not seen as being a particularly innovative contributor to work in 'Bloggs' disease' or 'Jones' disease' or 'Brown's disease'. I'm impossible to pigeonhole and I have an uncomfortable feeling that I'm not appreciated externally as much as I think I am, certainly by some people internally anyway. I get continuing requests to 'Please give a ten-lecture course on . . .', usually statistics for our postgraduate students. This stuff arrives if not weekly, then two or three times a year, but that's all local, so I don't have a thirteen- or fifteen-year life plan. I guess I don't want to stay where I am, doing what I am, for the next seventeen years until I'm sixty-five, and then quietly drop off the perch. I wouldn't at all mind switching into something else if an appropriate opportunity came along. That something else could only be to do with sport because of what I've done in that field, and at the moment there isn't anything looming on the horizon, and I'm not yet in a position to try and create it.

I'm drawn to sport because it combines three things which I've always enjoyed: physical exercise, competition and, to some extent, the outdoors. When I began doing the usual wheelchair things of table tennis and basketball, I gradually got rather bored. Every year at Stoke Mandeville you met the same people doing the same things in a small country town forty miles outside London, and I began to wonder, is this what it consists of? So I started looking more widely. Through an obscure contact, somebody in an office of the Sports Council asked me to take part in a week at Plas-y-Brenin in North Wales which is the Sports Council's Outdoor Activities Centre (now the National Centre for Mountain Activities). They were holding an outdoor adventure course for instructors of disabled people, and they wanted some disabled people to go along as guinea pigs. This had come about through the Disabled Sports Club which we'd developed at the university, but I was already beginning to feel uncomfortable with the concept of disabled people doing things together. So I went for this outdoor activities course, where I tried canoeing for the first time and enjoyed it enormously, although the weather was awful and it just poured with rain the whole time.

After that, I began to think not only about extending sports activities, about what else one could do, but also about the context in which they were done. Just before Christmas I came across an advertisement for Churchill fellowships and one of them was called Leisure and Recreational Procedure for the Disabled, so I applied. I got one, and went to the States to look at outdoor and adventure activities and at integration, and that I think was what finally made the scales drop from my eyes as far as disabled people in society were concerned. Here in Birmingham specifically, and in England generally then – possibly in the whole of Britain, let's not be nationalistic about this – there were still the swivelling eyeballs, and people staring at you in the street as you trundled along in your chair. The first morning in America, in Chicago, I was out on the pavement outside the hotel where the National Paraplegic Conference was taking place. I sort of wandered along the Chicago pavement, and people walked into me and didn't bat an eyelid. It wasn't that there were hundreds of wheelchairs out on the pavement at the time, because there weren't, it was as though you were nobody to be particularly remarked upon, you didn't present an unusual image. Do you remember one of the games we played as kids? You would stand beside a wall and press your arm hard against it, very hard, then you'd walk away from the wall and your arm would float up? Well, in Chicago it was as if I was floating, having been released from the pressure of everybody else's eyeballs. That was very interesting, nothing to do with sport specifically, although most of the rest of the time I was looking at sport, but that was one thing which hit me very strongly. It was the same more or less wherever you went in the States, nobody batted an eyelid.

I tried to get going on the sports side of things and I got injured training too hard – I did bits of sailing and canoeing up at the university's outdoor centre. That first morning in the States, I'd met the people who had organized the wheelchair bit of the Boston marathon, and this was happening in an integrated setting. How different from Stoke Mandeville, when the people who came to watch were always people from Aylesbury, and the local paper used to run a supplement on what everyone called the Goodwill Games, with 'heroic people doing wonderful things'. It was always really tacky stuff. We were segregated, of course and you never saw any able-bodied sports people there. Maybe one of them would come along to open it, but people who watch sport didn't go to Stoke, they'd go to Wembley or Lords or Crystal Palace or wherever. It seemed to me that, like mountains and Mohammed, you turn it the other way round and take the 'disabled sport activity' into the able-bodied setting so that people are forced to see, whether they want to or not. Of course this led on to marathons. Chris Brasher wrote an article in the *Observer* in the autumn of 1980, having just been to see the New York Marathon, saying how important it was that London had a marathon like this. I wrote back saying, 'Yes, I agree, and I hope there will be a wheelchair section.' This began a two-and-a-half-year campaign. In 1979 you were not allowed to run a marathon unless you were an AAA (Amateur Athletics Association) registered athlete – a bit like playing soccer in a local park team, you have to be registered with the regulating authority. In 1981, John Walker, a local guy here, decided he wanted to let anybody have a chance of running a marathon, so he instituted what was known as the People's Marathon, all of course done unofficially as far as the AAA were concerned. After the first London Marathon, Britain went mad on marathons and a number of us went and did them – I did two or three in 1981, four or five in 1982, six in 1983 and so on. One year, in 1983 or 1984, there were about 150 marathons in Britain. We just went mad. Most places found it something of a curiosity to have a wheelchair there, and most also let you dictate the terms under which you took part – i.e., letting you start the wheelchair in front, otherwise it would hit the ankles of people that were running. It took two and a half years to get a wheelchair section in the London Marathon, with me sitting in Birmingham beavering away writing to newspapers and to MPs, and discussing things with the GLC (Greater London Council). Eventually the IAAF (International Amateur Athletics Federation) were brought in by the GLC. Occasionally things appeared in the press, and eventually we got in, but the first year we were made to start at the back which was stupid. After that we were allowed to start at the front.

The really important thing, though, was that people could see a 'disabled sports event' actually taking place in tandem with an able-bodied sports event, to encourage a public perception that it was part of athletics and not specifically a disabled sport. It was just part of the whole spectrum of athletics. There are very few other contexts in which you can have that kind of concurrent participation. On an athletics track you can't have people in wheelchairs racing against people on legs, but what you can do, and what had happened by then, was that in an afternoon of athletics either at Crystal Palace or at the Alexander Stadium in Birmingham, there would be a wheelchair event. That's fine, you're putting a wheelchair event among the athletics public, so to speak, and that's a different model, but it's dictated by the nature of the activity. It's a bit like when the Basketball Association has its finals at Crystal Palace at the beginning of May: they have the boys' final at ten o'clock, the girls' final at twelve o'clock, the women's final at two o'clock, the wheelchair final at six o'clock, and the final at eight o'clock. But for road racing, the point is we had TV coverage and that's the crucial thing. Even now, when did you see the winter Paralympics? They weren't on live: the winter Paralympics were packaged into a one-hour programme and shown on Good Friday afternoon a fortnight after they'd finished. If you've got people in wheelchairs taking part in the same event as people running, the cameras will have to be very nifty to avoid showing a wheelchair at all during the four hours of transmission of the event. Now, of course, they don't avoid it, they actually focus in on things, and that's what it was all about.

I was inspired, originally, by the able-bodied organizers of the Boston Marathon. The year I went there, 1978, was the third year they'd included wheelchairs. That year they started the wheelchairs twenty minutes in front of everybody else, and the first wheelchair finished two minutes ahead of the first runner, so actually the distance between wheelchair and runner was decreasing. The proximity of the two made fantastic television, of course!

Nowadays you'd start the wheelchairs one minute in front, and they would finish half an hour or forty minutes ahead. That model, of what was originally just a running event, where the wheelchair participation becomes a part of the overall occasion, is such a simple model to follow, and it's an easy one to adopt in that context. I felt, given that we were going to have publicly televised marathons in London, that was a model that we should try and emulate. If you want to be cynical about it, it's leaching on somebody else's activity. I firmly believe, though, that it actually adds to the overall occasion and has pointed up the possibility of greater integration for people with a disability in able-bodied sports. How you can do it, and whether it's possible, depends on what the sport is. You can't have people in wheelchairs racing against somebody on the track on legs, not sensibly.

There have to be different categories, of course, and that has led on to a more extended and deeper reflection on the organizational structure of sport for people with a disability. It got me into dead trouble with Stoke Mandeville because I was arguing quite strongly against their restriction on participation to spinal-injury users only as distinct from wheelchair users in general. No amputees were allowed to participate for a long time. That's all settled down now, and amps are just as welcome as anybody else, you can cope with them under a suitable classification system.

Having watched from the side while people like Mike Oliver and Jenny Morris have achieved what they have, on what I'd call the sociology of disability, has been quite useful in pushing my thoughts along on where sport fits within the framework. Mike and Jenny have obviously queried, and I think rightly, why disabled people should always be seen as overcoming tremendous problems and achieving things despite their handicaps. It's always the medical model 'the disaster' and 'in spite of'. If you take three simple examples: Nelson Mandela has achieved what he has, not despite being black but because he is black; Germaine Greer achieved what she did, not despite being a woman but because she's a woman; Derek Jarman achieved what he did, not despite being gay but because he was gay. Therefore the public may have to think that at least some people with a disability have achieved what they have because of it, rather than in spite of it. Those models, which are obvious to everybody as soon as you say them, force you to look rather differently at disabled people, certainly at the individual level, and maybe generally as well.

Having discovered wheelchair road racing in America, I then went on to do that in a big way. I'd more or less dropped table tennis and basketball. I did quite a bit of canoeing in the late 1970s and early 1980s, and then got into sailing. I've also done winter sports, both competitively and recreationally. Winter sports in the generic sense, of course: I've tried cross-country sledding but it was much too much like hard work; I've tried ice-sledge racing which is much too much like hard work; and I've tried ice hockey which is hard work but not if you play in goal because you sit there and try to fill the goal! I've never won any awards for sport.

I was picked for the team for the Lillehammer Olympics, but I got an injured shoulder so I couldn't play. I've had a selection in wheelchair racing for the marathon in Japan in 1984, various selections for winter sports activities, both ice-sledge racing and sledge hockey, and at one scary stage a downhill sledge. If you're Linford Christie, you know that you're at the pinnacle of tens if not hundreds of thousands of people who run 100 metres. The same cannot be said for the selection in winter sports events for disabled people in this country. At the moment, the numbers taking part are very small. That's true internationally as well, although as people have developed new kinds of equipment, particularly in the winter-sports field, the numbers overseas, particularly of Continental Europeans taking part, are far greater than here. Winter sports generically is a very small area of activity for disabled people from this country, and whilst it was very nice to go to Switzerland to play sledge hockey, I couldn't think actually how hard I'd struggled to get this far and how many people I'd clambered over, because I hadn't.

I've never been to the summer Paralympics. I've been to individual European championships or world championships, mostly when they've been in a very embryonic state, not just as far as people from this country are concerned but as far as the organization of the event itself it concerned, and therefore there have been relatively few people taking part. It's not, for example, like the summer Paralympics which has probably thirty or forty countries that play wheelchair basketball at least. Well, the winter sports is nowhere near that far along, and probably never will be. Far fewer people take part in the winter Olympics than the summer Olympics and far fewer countries, and that's even more the case on the disabled side.

Before the accident I never thought about disabilities. It's not been as awful as you might have thought. If I was trying to put myself back into the legs of an able-bodied person nowadays, or went back twenty-two years, if I'd been asked about it beforehand, I might have thought it would be awful and dreadful, but it's not.

I wouldn't go as far as I believe Mike Oliver has and say it was the best thing that ever happened to me. If I were offered my legs back, I'd have them like a shot, but that doesn't mean that I'm going to spend my whole life moping and saying 'Oh dear, I do wish I could walk, I do wish, I do wish . . .' I'd be a miserable bugger if I did that all day. So although I can envisage it theoretically, of course it's not practical.

I think my biggest achievement since disability has been getting a wheelchair section in the London Marathon. It sounds a bit trivial but it wasn't, I can tell you, it took a lot of aggro. I suppose one of the other things, which again is on the side, strictly outside work, is to help the Sports Council focus more on the place of disabled sport in Britain. In particular, I've been responsible for pushing forward an integration thrust, trying to get the able-bodied governing bodies of sport more interested in disability, not in itself, but in disabled people of all kinds doing their particular sports. Professionally, well, I'm just a jobbing epidemiologist. I'm having some interesting experiences at the moment trying to develop a management structure for the Department of Public Health and Epidemiology, which has never had one. We have about forty staff and for the last eighteen months we've had devolved departmental budgets. You cannot bumble on just doing things as they've always been done when you have what amounts to a Sword of Damocles hanging above you, so I've been trying to develop a management structure, which is a culture shock for everybody, including me. That's been professionally stretching, particularly since I have no formal training in this field at all, and also because I've never experienced it, because the department has never been run like that. We've not finished yet, either, as it's a process of continuous evolution: the external requirements on you change and increase, and it's not for me to judge how well I've done. Some people at work think things are a lot better than they were, which is nice, but we recognize that the more you try and do, the more you realize what a shambles it is.

People constantly want to know, 'How do you manage to cope?' 'How long did it take you to adjust?' In everything I do I try to challenge the 'tragic but brave' stereotype of disability. It amounts to unthinking discrimination and I try to turn these questions back. I've got slightly less harsh in my reactions to such questions over the last few years, but they are still silly questions, they're unanswerable. The reason for being less harsh is that if you get really stroppy with people, they go away and think, 'Gosh, isn't he all screwed up?'

Paradoxically the 'talking out' of the Civil Rights (Disabled Persons) Bill in the House of Commons in May 1994 may have the effect of ensuring that the government actually does something. It'll be a curious outcome if that's what happens, but it certainly has raised the profile of the issue of civil rights. I've met the Minister concerned, Nick Scott, and actually like him as a man. I think he's been a very empathetic Minister but I don't think he's so machiavellian as to have fitted this up in order to raise the level of government commitment. I think it was a cock-up, it was a cover-up rather than a plot to make things even better than the Bill itself would have done, but nevertheless it may yet result in something concrete coming out from a not very happy series of events. At one level I would almost like to get hold of the politicians in this country and shake them, and make them try and see sense. Mum apparently used to say when I was in my teens that she thought I would go into politics, but I'm too much of an anarchist to subscribe rigorously to any party discipline.

I certainly encounter discrimination, but not active discrimination. It's more that I can't get into places. I'm prevented from going to the Hexagon Theatre in the Midlands Arts Centre because there are three steps up into it and two steps down inside or something so they won't let me in. I've been in once – it was several years ago now, and I don't think they realized what they were doing – but I've missed several things that I've wanted to go to and I think next time I will just offer to bum my way up the stairs. The wheelchair is perceived as an obstruction, a hazard and a danger if you're sitting there in a seat. Years ago I went to *The Ring* at the Hippo (the Birmingham Hippodrome theatre), performed by English National Opera. In the mid to late 1970s they let wheelchairs in for nothing. I've been there a number of times since, and at one stage you weren't allowed to sit in your wheelchair in a gangway in the aisle because you were defined as a fire risk. But if you got out of your wheelchair and sat in the seat at the end of a row and your wheelchair was tucked away up the back somewhere, that was fine. Now that is a bananas perception, because you block half the row from getting out, never mind not being able to get out yourself. I've had various spats about that, at a local level. I've also had spats about the provision of wheelchair toilets in motorway service stations. I once wrote a long and detailed letter to Jill Knight, MP for Birmingham, Edgbaston, about trying to sit on the loo at Charnock Richards Service Station on the M6. At that stage, the only so-called wheelchair loo was just an ordinary loo with two diagonal handrails fixed inside with an inward-opening door which you couldn't close when you got inside in the wheelchair. I invited her to think how she would feel if she was invited to defecate in public, which is what it came down to. Things have changed there now, they've designed and built a proper wheelchair loo.

In principle, you can argue it doesn't matter a stuff whether these places provide wheelchair facilities or not, though they should do so in accordance with the 1970 Act. The only people that can put up notices on motorways are the Ministry of Transport, and they shouldn't put up notices on big blue signs with a wheelchair sign, if there isn't a facility there or it's inadequate. That was my line of argument, but I think it's a drop in the ocean. I was probably just another of these irritating people writing but eventually the message begins to get through. I can't talk about discrimination in employment because I haven't experienced it; I've been unusual and very lucky in that respect.

One obvious area of passive discrimination is transport. Last year we went to Barcelona for a long weekend and I did something that I haven't done for twenty-one years – I got on a public service bus and paid a fare. As you might imagine, it was an astonishing feeling. It was also bloody uncomfortable: all the buses from Barcelona Airport to the middle of town are low-floor buses. (I'm told this is also true now of many of the buses from the middle of London out to London Airport.) Arriving at Barcelona, you get on a low-floor bus and then people come and struggle past you and lean on top of you and so on. Who would choose to travel that way? But I actually paid a fare and what a kick it gave me! I would love to be able to trundle down the road and hop on a bus and go into town. Every time I go to town I either have to drive or I go from the railway station which now at last has a lift. For the first sixteen years of its existence, the newly built university railway station didn't have a lift.

I also object to petrol stations where they won't come and serve you, and to other people looking at me. If other people stare at me, I think they've got a problem, that's the only sensible attitude to take. If they stare at me because they think I'm peculiar, then it's they who've got the problem, not me.

Things are changing, though. There are more ramps – not so much ramps as approaches to buildings so that they don't require ramps: you have a gradually rising thing with a flush bit at the top. There's the perception that people should all come in the same entrance: you don't have separate entrances for disabled people, which is segregating, labelling, stigmatizing, and you don't need them anyway. Of course, we've got a problem with old buildings, because you can't always have a wheelchair going in the front door like everybody else. I've never tried to get into St Paul's Cathedral, but I've seen pictures and know there's a flight of steps up at the front. I don't know how people in wheelchairs do get into St Paul's, but I'm not sure that putting a ramp up the front is appropriate. Simply because people in wheelchairs can't get up into the

Bloody Tower or the White Tower (at the Tower of London), I am dead certain that they should not therefore be closed, which is some people's reaction – that if disabled people can't get into places, they should not be part of the public domain. I disagree.

There are things I don't do, but I don't think that's specifically because of the disability. They're mostly on the sporting side: I won't go hang-gliding or diving, for instance. They're both things I would like to have done, but I haven't got the bottle; I don't think that's to do with the disability, I think I would have felt like that beforehand.

I met my wife when I was hoiked into the local hospital at four o'clock in the morning with very severe gut pain which turned out to be gallstones. She was nursing on the ward that I was put on, a medical ward despite my having had a surgical operation. The nursing was very good, and Caroline was one of the nurses. After I got out I asked her if she would come round for a meal. She did, and things went from there, very quickly actually.

Caroline could probably tell you how she's coped with my disability better than I can. I guess she's become more aware of the issues about disability than she might have done. She finds me difficult to deal with at times because I'm a fairly forceful character but then that's what I'm like, and I don't think that's specifically to do with disability. Both our lives have changed somewhat, hers rather more than mine, partly because I stayed in the same place, and she moved in here so it was a bigger change for her than it was for me, but she's a fairly independent sort. If you look outside, all the stuff on the patio is her doing, the cold frame, and all the plants. She's got an allotment which is about twice the size of the surface area of this flat. We hardly ever buy potatoes, and no onions or garlic, she grows it all. That's what she wants to do, actually, have a smallholding and do it properly with animals as well, but you've got to win the football pools or something like that to be able to get into that position.

If she could do it, if we could afford to buy one, I'd be happy. In the first instance it depends how much you get, doesn't it? £250,000 used to be the top amount but it isn't enough for me to retire on. It's enough for her to retire on, and for us to get a smallholding for her to work on, but you need more than that, given that I've got another seventeen years of full-time work and heaven knows how many more years after that. You need more than that if you are going to retire comfortably now.

At the moment, Caroline does most of the housework. She's employed three days a week, and the other two days, if you like, are for her to do house stuff and her own thing – the allotment. I do virtually all the washing up, and that's my lot. She does the cleaning, the cooking, the shopping and, when it comes to it, the decorating. You saw the bathroom, well, she did that entirely, she redecorated that from scratch. OK, she didn't put the bath in or the basin, and the plumbing was left unaltered, but she did all the surfaces. I'm not always so indolent, because when she was working five days a week and doing nights which used to be a seven-night stretch, she was absolutely knackered, I did almost everything: the shopping, the cooking, the washing up, but not the cleaning. That I loathe, it's much more difficult for me to do than for her and it actually seems a sensible division of labour to me, but then it would, wouldn't it, because it's sexist and so on. I do all the driving as well. I know that's not housework, and she has her own car, but if we go anywhere it's me that does the driving. We try to share things out as evenly as possible.

I can't tell what I would have been like coping with the practicalities of life if I hadn't become disabled. Before I became disabled I was living in a flat, cooking, cleaning, washing up, and doing that adequately, I thought, it certainly wasn't a tip. Clearly my disability has made it more difficult to do some things like the cleaning: trundling around a vacuum is more difficult in a wheelchair than it is on legs, and therefore it tends to be something that I would avoid if I possibly could. Before Caroline turned up I did do it because there wasn't anybody else to do it. I suppose I could have hired a cleaning lady, but I chose not to.

Mum was a bit shocked when I first became disabled, but she's coped very well. I remember one occasion when I was still living down with her at Evesham. We went out into the middle of town and I wanted to push up the steep hill from the bridge across the Avon. I was just out of hospital and hadn't developed the kind of arm- and shoulder-strength that I have since. I insisted on pushing up it, with her walking beside me, and she said she saw people staring across at her, clearly wondering why on earth she didn't offer to help. She found that very difficult to cope with, but it was other people's reactions that bothered her, rather than me. I think she's coped with this remarkably well, it's not a change that anybody would wish on someone. I think she feels I've become almost as stroppy and opinionated as Dad (who died when I was eleven) was. Well, not quite, he did things much more his own way.

My friends from the climbing club were the people that I socialized with most before my accident. I didn't have a social circle in Birmingham as such, and still don't really. Some of them were a little bit wary, did I really want to see them again, did I really want to have any involvement with mountains. This was my perception, nobody actually said this, but I'm sure the feeling was, would I really want to have anything to do with the mountains that had done this dreadful thing to me. One of the climbing club cottages is about five miles from where the spinal unit was, so there were lots of opportunities for people to come and visit, and lots of people did. They'd roll in on a Sunday evening at five o'clock after they had a weekend's walking or climbing, and that was good. I'm just the same person I have always been. I don't go rock climbing any longer, but I spend a lot of weekends with people in the climbing club in North Wales or the Lake District or Derbyshire, and at New Year for the last twelve or thirteen years almost every year, I've been away with a bunch of people and we stay at the same place: they go downhill ski-ing or walking, and I go cross-country sledding.

I'm sure growing old will create more physical problems. My shoulders particularly are in a dicky state, partly because I've hammered them. I don't hammer them so much now but I'm sure arthritis could develop, because of the lifting and turning. There is also a potential skin problem, too, because the skin and the tissues underneath get more fragile as one ages, and there's a much greater potential for skin damage if you're sixty than if you're twenty. The healing time would be correspondingly much longer, as well. But these are theoretical concepts at the moment.

I've just got to be very careful. I won't be able to do that much about the arthritis if it comes. So far as the skin is concerned, I do believe you can protect yourself to a very great extent with all the cushions there are nowadays. Not that I've got one of them, but I would if it came to it. One thing I've never had is pressure sores. I've had scrapes on my skin, but I've never had a pressure sore, and certainly for a paraplegic it's totally unnecessary, as you can avoid them by having a decent cushion. If you can't afford a decent cushion, you can avoid sores by lifting yourself up for fifteen seconds, every fifteen minutes. In forty years' time I might not be able to get away with just that. It was something that was drilled into me at the spinal unit. The new cases who were up and about, but who weren't doing any lifting, were taken into what we called the leper colony. This was the ward with real live patients who had pressure sores to various extents. I never went down there, I don't think I could have coped with seeing that. The worst thing you can do to help develop pressure sores is sit still, drink lots of alcohol and get fat. If you eat lots of fatty foods, you'll get fat and that's no good to man nor beast. I think you must have a certain amount of sense on diet. I love wine and drink lots of wine but in moderation; I mean I'm not a two bottles a night man, I probably get through about a bottle a week. You have to be sensible. Certainly since I had the shoulder problems, I've had to be slightly more careful about what I eat: I can't burn it all off in very sharp exercise because it will wreck my shoulders. If you are moderately sensible – though people's perception of what's sensible varies somewhat – you will be OK. I think a certain amount of exercise is obviously sensible, and how you choose to take it is very much up to you. Some people choose to take it by thrashing around in wheelchairs and getting horribly fit that way. Nowadays my exercise tends to be just pushing around in the wheelchair, not for its own sake but going places, going to work, going shopping or trundling around mountains.

I'm lucky in that I've never actually had to move house. I was in the university hall of residence for ten years all told when I came out of hospital. I bought my present flat seven years after I started in the hall of residence, and, both while I was there and since I've left, the university has made further adaptations to make the whole place more accessible, particularly for wheelchair users. In terms of accommodation, we're specifically talking about wheelchair users rather than visually handicapped or hearing-impaired people, but I thought I should look for somewhere of my own. It seemed a sensible thing to do, to have somewhere in case I got kicked out of the hall of residence or something. It was just an ordinary advertisement in the paper, and after looking at about three places, this was the only one I could sensibly, realistically, get into. There is no ramp up the front, but at the moment I don't need it because I can bounce up the step. In fact for a time there was a ramp round the back for the dustbin men to take the big skips off, but that disappeared years ago when they changed the fitting on the skips. The only adaptation I've had done to the flat is to have the loo door taken off. It used to open back against the loo which made it impossible to get at, so I had it taken off and put a screen up there. Caroline couldn't cope with this when she came along, so she put the door on the other way round.

I work on the ground floor of the medical school. The main entrance is up a flight of steps, but the whole thing is on a slight rise and fall both side to side and back to front, and at one place there is a flat entrance so I just come in there straight on to the ground floor. There are minor problems over reaching up to put stuff on overhead projectors which I sometimes can't reach, and I certainly can't reach to write on them because they're basically at head, forehead or hairline level. I can't actually see what's on them, nor can I see the placement of an overhead slide on the thing. I can only guess what's showing up by seeing what's on the screen behind and certainly couldn't write anything. That's a fairly minor technical detail, but as far as the rest is concerned, it's OK.

Birmingham is not a centre for the management of spinal injuries and therefore there's nobody who is an expert in that respect locally. The kind of management I received at the spinal unit as an outpatient was, to begin with, very authoritarian: you were not put down, but you were managed as though you were a child, and that was the characteristic of the particular clinician concerned. That kind of management has changed somewhat, and now I feel you're treated much more as a partner, as someone to contribute to your own care rather than them doing it all for you or indeed them telling you what to do. I guess that's partly a change of time and certainly a change of consultants as well. In terms of my professional contact with other doctors, they're contacting me for my expertise in statistics and epidemiology, and study design, and nothing to do with the wheelchair, so in that respect the wheelchair is a bit of an irrelevance. I certainly don't feel that I'm being molly-coddled or patronized by anyone who comes to see me on those grounds. It's sometimes a bit of a shock if they don't know, if they ring me up because they've been given my name by somebody else, and say, 'Can I come and see you?' As they come through the door, most of them cope with it very well, but I deliberately don't say anything such as 'Oh, you didn't realize I was in a wheelchair, did you?' There's no point, because that makes it artificial, as though I'm trying to score points off them. Nevertheless, I do occasionally notice the double take and, at the same time, how well they adapt to it, and how well they adapt to their own surprise.

One practical problem which is unchanging is bowel management – every evening, manual evacuation. At the hospital, things were done in the mornings and you're relatively inactive in hospital, not zipping around all day, and so it was every two days. I couldn't sustain that, so I had to switch to every morning and the problem with the morning is that, if you get up late, then everything is rushed. You've always got more time in the evenings, in addition to which you've been sitting up all day rather than lying down for eight hours or so. I've switched to every evening, and that's what I do now.

Going away or going on a long flight, things have to be timed, you have to be very careful. We went to Australia and New Zealand last year, and it wasn't a problem; it's just a question of making sure that you don't do a thirty-six hour non-stop flight which would cause problems, but you can always take medication to stop things shifting through so fast. I did that when I went to Japan, but actually I didn't take any when we went to Australia and New Zealand; we were breaking the journey at Singapore, it was about a twenty-four hour day. There is a degree of latitude of about five or six hours either way which is helpful, provided you are sensible with what you eat. I love raw cauliflower, but I can only eat a very little of it before it has disastrous effects. I love rhubarb as well, but I can only eat so much of it. For bladder control, I just wear a sheath, a condom, and have done ever since the start. I'm still on the old system. I've still got to change to the self-adhesive systems which are around nowadays. I've got rather tender skin, and the consultant at the spinal unit said 'That looks a bit fierce' about the glue on the self-adhesive sheaths. I've got to start trying them, however, because the old system just won't be available any longer at some point. That works OK, and maybe once a year, once every eighteen months, something splits and I get wet, but it's never happened away from either work or home. It's very, very rare, so I think in practical terms the management of that is as successful as it could be.

I can't pretend to be au fait with the latest research into regeneration of the spinal cord. I read in the American sports magazine *Sports and Spokes* the ads saying, 'Come and have your paralysed muscles regenerated, and we'll get you walking again', and I wrinkle my nose, not with displeasure or distaste but with scepticism. The consultant in charge of the spinal unit when I was in said he thought that a 'cure' might come but it would be thirty years at least, and it would come through biochemistry. I think we may have moved on and not a cure, but a way of overcoming the neurological deficit may come through electronic signalling, but we're probably still thirty years away from that as well. Six years ago, I had syringomyelia which is a spinal cyst which works up through the spinal cord. It gradually knocks off various things, first of all sensory usually, then motor. I was operated on in Smethwick, the local neurosurgical centre. Opposite me in the same ward was another guy with a spinal injury who was a member of the International Spinal Research Trust. He was convinced that he was going to be walking in five years' time. His five years were up last December, and I don't have any contact with him, but I think he'll have been severely disappointed. He had the faith of the true believer that the ISRT was going to find the answer, but they haven't so far.

I once saw a film about a technique by which black boxes are implanted to connect muscles internally. They don't help with walking and getting around in the sense that I think is practically useful. If you live near a shopping centre with flat floors everywhere, and you really want to be upright and move around, then you can do so using the implant technique, but actually it's not a realistic way of getting about over the kind of ground that I cover for example between here and work in the wheelchair, or the kind of ground that I would want to go on if I was away at weekends with the climbing club. I know somebody who wrote articles saying 'the dream of all paraplegics to be able to walk again is now nearly realized'. There is a belief held, possibly quite widely, by the medical profession and by others that it's what wheelchair users want most of all to do. I don't think it is. I mean if I was told, 'You can walk like you used to', I'd say yes, please, but it isn't like that.

What's on offer is not walking like able-bods walk, it's walking in a jerky stilted motion with electrodes stuck to you, wires hanging off you, and black boxes strung round your waist, with a zimmer frame in front of you. That's not meant to be critical about people who do use zimmer frames routinely, without all the electronics, but it's not walking in any realistic sense as a means of getting about.

It seems to me the scientists are doing a disservice by raising people's hopes to an extent that I think is dreadful. It says something generally about the psychological rehabilitation of those people before they left the spinal unit. If those are the ambitions they left the spinal unit with, the spinal unit in my view has not done its job properly. You could say this guy's a terribly difficult character and he won't listen to anything we tell him, in which case he needs more psychology. (You could say it's just a group of scientists who are practising their evil arts upon us, the psychologists rather than the physicists or the electronic engineers.) Even without the limitations of no steps and bumpy uneven pavements and so on, it's a lot more energy-efficient getting around in a wheelchair than on crutches, and much easier.

I wonder about people who design things for disabled people. A small example that I've come across is the supermarket shopping trolley: somebody designed this version that attaches to the front of a wheelchair, and you go eight or nine feet long along the aisle with this thing rigidly attached to the wheelchair in front of you. Well, that's all very well, provided you don't want to turn round. They were quite a fad about ten years ago. It isn't all that easy trundling an ordinary supermarket trolley along because you know how wayward they are; and pushing the wheelchair along at the same time isn't that easy even for me. You can't reach as much as you'd like to and you have to have an able bod there if you want to reach high, or at least somebody to ask. But if you are locked into something that's eight feet long, you can't turn round and say, 'Blast, I've forgotten that, I'll just go back.' That all seems to me a bit of a nonsense, but I haven't seen one being used recently.

Transport is changing too. I've got photographs from 1978 from my trip to the States of the low-floor bus which was just being developed there, and was seen as a solution to transport, certainly city transport, for disabled people. If you're going to buy a bus, why not buy a low-floor bus, but there were technology problems with them. People have got over that now, they can build low-floor buses successfully, and they don't need any more maintenance than ordinary buses, so why not make all buses low-floored? Trains are a slightly different matter. Because you have to have a gap between the floor of an express train and a platform level – simply because they go through platforms at high speed – the physics of it apparently forbid you having the floor too flush to the platform. If they're too flush, there's no room for air to spill around, and you end up either ripping the carriage or ripping the platform to pieces. There will always be problems about trains. Some of the newer ones are actually rather lower and closer to the platform than the old ones, but it varies because platforms are not all at a uniform height. I think my best experience on a train was in eastern Switzerland where they are narrow gauge, only one metre, so there's not an awful lot of room. They don't put disabled people in the middle of all the carriages, but in the guard's van, opposite the guard's section, they've got a separate cubicle-type thing for wheelchair users. There's room for two wheelchair users or one wheelchair user and somebody else with them in their own heated section beside a large picture window. OK, it's private, but the able bod can wander up and down the main train, and of course the scenery is beautiful. We were on honeymoon when we experienced that, so maybe it was coloured by the glow, but it was very well done, and shipping people down from one train to another was very well done too.

I think the move to make all taxis wheelchair accessible is a good one, but how many people can afford to travel by taxi? It's public transport that needs to be accessible, and low-floor buses should be mandatory everywhere. Trains I've talked about. With aeroplanes, they're trying to shoe-horn as many people as possible into as small a space as possible. It's interesting that in Prague, about a month ago, the attendant staff for the wheelchair were actually very good. They stood back and waited until I asked them to do things, they didn't rush up and grab hold of me and push me and pull me which I might have expected. I know it's a horrible prejudice to have, but I wouldn't have expected them to be as enlightened as that. They did much better than the staff in Barcelona quite honestly, who nearly dropped me coming down the aircraft steps and that was after Barcelona had had the Paralympics.

I actually went to Barcelona three times within about six months. I went to the Olympics with a friend whose wife was captain of the British women's hockey team, just as a private citizen. Then I was sent back a month later by the Sports Council for about six days to see the Paralympics, and then we went on a long weekend in February last year.

People offer me help rather less often than they used to, and I suspect that's because they've come round to realizing that wheelchair users are capable of doing things, that they're not as incapable as they might once have seemed. If people do offer to help, you mustn't snap their heads off even if it is the tenth time that day that you've received such an offer, and you don't want any of it. It may be the first time not only that day, but that year, that they've offered help to anybody, it may have taken them a lot of courage to get round to doing so, and if you snap their head off, they'll feel aggrieved and they may not offer help to anybody ever again. But one thing people offering help should never do is take hold of the wheelchair and start pushing it, pulling it, or lifting it without asking or being asked.

It is quite impossible for me to say how I've coped emotionally with my disability. I went to the national games at Stoke Mandeville one week after I was discharged, and there were people being presented with medals for having been to all twenty-five national paraplegic games. I said to myself, 'I'll be here in twenty-five years' time getting one of those medals'. The realization developed, as I found myself getting drawn more and more into it, that there was a wheelchair world and a real world. The wheelchair world seemed to be, socially and recreationally, entirely taken up with other people in wheelchairs. It was a shock to the system to get to America and find out that even at the paraplegic conference, people in wheelchairs didn't only talk with people in wheelchairs, they socialized with able bods as well. One shouldn't get totally sucked into it, and let oneself be completely circumscribed and limited to socializing with other people in wheelchairs. One should never be defined by one's disability.

I think people with disabilities should maintain or develop contacts and friendships to do with things and activities that they're interested in. For example, I have social contacts with people in the wheelchair racing world; we all happen to have a disability, but it's the wheelchair racing that is the focus of interest. I have contacts and social activities with people in the sailing club, and I'm the only wheelchair user there at the moment, although there have been the odd one or two in the past. But the common interest is sailing and all the other people who walk around on legs see me as a sailor, not as a disabled person. I think it's crucially important for living a full life; or it gives you a fuller life than if your whole world is defined by the wheelchair. I think that to let that happen is a mistake.

I think this country needs an Anti-Discrimination Act. It may not produce financial benefits, and that's not what Roger Berry's Bill was about, it was about seeing people with a disability as citizens with full rights who are part of the society, and who not only contribute to the society, but have rightful expectations of society.

I think changes in the law would have the potential to be very successful. The Americans with Disabilities Act is obviously a template, a model which could be used in this country, though clearly in the short term at least it's not going to be. The area of access is an obvious one, but employment is also crucial. I've argued in the past that you need a tripod of things to enable you to lead what you might call a successful life: you need somewhere to live; you need some way of getting about; and you need something to do. Now the something to do doesn't necessarily have to be paid employment, it could be voluntary work.

People with spinal injuries can promote awareness of spinal injury in two ways. You can either look at it from a preventative point of view or a 'How do we manage it now we've got it' view. For a preventative perspective, you need to look at those groups in society that are most at risk, or those people into whom you can din messages that will stay when they come to be of the relevant risk ages. For the latter in particular, you're talking about school kids. Obviously you get at school kids by giving talks or whatever about the hazards, although you have to be careful not to scare them by leaving them with the impression that they mustn't go outside the front door, because that would be extremely limiting. But that's a different slant from how you should generate awareness of the issues and problems that people with spinal injury have. In some respects they're no different from those of anyone in wheelchairs – the things I've just been talking about, accessible accommodation, accessible transport, non-discrimination in employment and so on. I don't think it's appropriate to try and raise people's consciousness about skin problems, sex problems, bladder problems, bowel problems, the things that are more specific to people with spinal injury. I think in some respects the things that one might promote are actually generic across a wide diagnostic range of disabilities, certainly in terms of what facilities and services are needed. Prevention is a more specific thing, and I think that can be targeted to some extent, though obviously not completely. About a fortnight ago, a group of people who had broken their necks playing rugby had a meeting at Twickenham to talk about prevention, about how to stop it from happening to other people. It's done within the context of the Rugby Football Union, brought together by the current president of the RFU who's very keen on prevention. Because of the club system, there's an organizational structure for getting messages out to a small – in population terms – but nevertheless at-risk group.

Raising the awareness of the public about the needs of people with spinal injury is tricky. You can put it on television programmes, but people often find disability a turn-off. You can write articles in newspapers, local big-wig disabled people can get messages in local newspapers and become local celebrities. We have so many channels of communication in the broadest sense of the term, fighting for our attention. I mean, how many of the television programmes you saw last year have stuck in your mind as 'Really tremendous, I can really remember that'? Four channels, plus all the satellite channels, plus radio, plus all the print media – I don't think it's realistic to expect a generic raising of public awareness. I don't think that's possible any longer, if indeed it ever was.

Feeding people with particular problems into soaps is a way that's been successful, I think there's no doubt about that. It could be somebody with a visual handicap or somebody with cerebral palsy, and just putting them in the programme as part of the routine, that gets people's attention and raises awareness far more I would think than any special programme. In a soap, we have characters who are seen regularly. I don't watch the TV soaps, to me they are a waste of time, but millions of people do.

If you were to show people with disabilities being demonstrably discriminated against in soaps, that will actually make people think. They may not come to the right conclusions but it's likely to make them think, that's one way. At a national level, you have to lobby, use political influence, Steve Bradshaw and people having lunch with MPs and so on, occasionally the 'big bang' demonstration like the one in London about two years ago where people chained themselves to buses or sat down in front of buses because the buses weren't accessible. Of course the police don't know how to move disabled people: do you pick them up the way they were picked up in the Ban the Bomb demonstrations in the 1960s, or what do you do with them? All this occasions a degree of public embarrassment, but you can't do it continually, because people don't have the psychological energy to keep that sort of thing going day after day. Even if they did, the TV people would soon get very bored with it, and they would go away.

So a certain amount can be done locally through action groups about access for instance, but I'm not sure how much can be done at a national level in terms of public awareness. I think it's getting at what I call the opinion formers, and for that more than anything you have to get to your local council or MP, and do pressure group work.

I don't think Caroline and I are very adventurous about holidays. Apart from last year which was a splurge on Australia and New Zealand, we tend to stick to Europe. I've absolutely no desire to go to North America again, I've been there two or three times, and it doesn't really interest me, which is awful really. Well, I'd quite like to go to Yellowstone and Grand Teton and to Yosemite and possibly Oregon and Washington State, but I'm not really interested in going to Washington DC, and am certainly not interested in going to Disneyland. We tend to go where I can drive because we sleep in the van: it acts as a camper van and so it's simply a question of finding a camp site. In Europe now there is a proliferation of camp sites with wheelchair-accessible loos, there are hundreds of them, although numbers vary in different countries. France is among the best equipped of the main European countries. Germany has got quite a lot, Switzerland very many fewer, Italy is OK in the north and west but less so in the south,

Austria is OK. We're going to eastern Switzerland this year. Holland is probably the best of all but we're not interested in going there.

What we have developed is going away on short weekend breaks. We have one main holiday a year, and go on a couple of short weekend breaks. That's a question of finding out whether the hotel is accessible, because we fly rather than drive, and I just do that by telephone, and keep my fingers crossed. We went on a short weekend break to Amsterdam: we were told the hotel was wheelchair accessible, but it turned out there were three steps up to the front. I wouldn't have expected that of Amsterdam, though inside it was all right. They said they always have staff available so you could always be picked up. There are places I want to go to. I want to go to Tierra del Fuego and I want to go to Alaska, I want to go to Baffin Island, I want to go to Concordia in the Karakoram just below K2, and I'd like to go to the Sahara. These tend to be remote places, as you can see, but I haven't seriously sorted out a system to enable me to get to them and have a sensible holiday there. I don't expect I'll get to all of them.

Caroline and I have talked about having children. Spinal injury makes it rather difficult and we decided that given the low probability of success and the difficulties with the procedures required, these together probably outweigh the wish that we might have for kids. It doesn't distress me, although it may do in twenty years' time when I realize finally, intellectually or emotionally, that I don't have a son and heir. That's a regret, but there are a lot of regrets.

I've been dead lucky having somewhere to live and something to do. I've had the resources to buy my own transport, and I've been lucky in finding a partner who's prepared to put up with my somewhat stroppy way of going about things. I'm lucky in that I'm a member of the Sports Council. This came about partly through having written and talked about the Stoke Mandeville exclusivity to spinal injury and having written stuff for the officer in the Sports Council. About five and a half years ago, Colin Moynihan (the then Minister for Sport) was getting together a group to look at the organization of disabled sport, and I guess they got in touch with the Sports Council officer concerned with this area to ask if he had any names of people to put forward. I think my name was slipped in sideways that way, so I joined this group. Then, halfway through the life of that group, Colin was changing the Sports Council and cutting it down, and he asked me if I'd be on it. There's a sort of statutory disabled person on the Sports Council, the same way that there is a statutory woman or a statutory ethnic minority person . . . It's not literally by statute, but there has to be a perception that someone with this particular area of expertise is a member, and I happen to be the 'statutory' disabled person at the moment. That's not said cynically at all. I'm not in any formal sense a representative, though I am seen as representing the interests of a particular group. But if you talked to any of us on the Council who could be seen to represent one of these interests, we'd all say that, at the end, when we leave, if that's all we're seen to have done, been involved with, just this group, then we'd have failed. You have to be involved with all the Council's work, not just a small, sectional interest. Anyway, I've been a member since October 1988, and we're in the middle of 1994. It's given me a tremendous insight into the organizational structure of sport in Britain. It's developed my expertise at chairing committees hugely, because I chair about three of the sub-committees as well as contributing to the main debates of the Council and this has been very very useful on a professional level as well. Although it's not my profession as such, the expertise or the skills of chairing committees are to some extent generic, and I've been able to take them into work and use them at work in a way which I wouldn't have developed in the same way or to the same extent if I hadn't had the opportunity on the Council. It's a precarious kind of existence because it's dependent on ministerial diktat – when your time's up, if the minister doesn't like you or thinks you've done enough, off you go.

We have a fixed term of office and eighteen months' time is the next time I'm up. It's been an interesting time in the life of the Sports Council because of all sorts of imminent and impending administrative changes to the structure, so I've been right up to date with that. The other thing is the content, which is actually completely different from anything I do at work and so it makes a wonderful change.

My piece of advice to other people in a comparable situation would be to try not to be bitter, even if it's not your fault and you don't have any compensation. I know two or three people to whom that happened, but try not to be bitter because it doesn't do you any good in the long run. It doesn't help you. Yes, it's a crying shame, and there's the 'why me?' business but there's always that. When I was in hospital somebody had a spinal cyst on the spinal cord which rendered him paraplegic: why him? If you sit around doing the 'why me?' business you'll end up in the 'personal tragedy' model of disability, which isn't a very positive way of living the rest of your life. You have to try to think positively, you know, 'Go placidly from this place . . .' and don't always just sit and moan and so on. You can still have a good life even if you think it's despite, rather than because of, the disability.

Stephen Bradshaw

Stephen Bradshaw was born in 1941. He is the executive director of the Spinal Injuries Association and has received the OBE. He sustained his spinal injury in 1967 in a diving accident. He lives in London.

In 1967, when I was twenty-five, I took a snap holiday, no insurance or anything sensible like that. We took a night flight out to Malta, then on to Gozo, to stay with a group of friends in a typical local stone house in a village called Gharb. The owner called it a villa, but it was an old farmer's house where all the animals used to be kept on the ground floor. There were outside staircases. It was wonderfully primitive, with just a tap out in the street, no running water or bathroom, so it was a young person's place. We spent our time dive-bombing the flies because they were just colossal and bit like mules! It was young people rushing round doing things, and we didn't bother to eat until the evening at six o'clock or so. We went swimming nearly every day at this beautiful sandy beach called Ramala Bay where, in the good old days, the Greeks and St Paul were said to have landed, and so it had all those wonderful associations. We looked at some amazing archaeological sites where they were excavating artefacts dating from before Christ.

Anyway I took a bet to pull down an outhouse – a sort of shed in the courtyard, made of huge stone blocks. The only tools were a chisel and a hammer, so there I was, slaving away in the hot sun. Eventually the demolition was done and, though completely exhausted, I won my bet. Then we all piled into the car and went down to the beach. I was larking around in a shallow area where I'd dived before – it was only about four feet deep at most – and I did this superb rugby tackle on my girlfriend. Unfortunately I hit the bottom before I crashed into her legs, and lost consciousness for a few seconds. By the time I surfaced, I had regained consciousness, but she ducked me and swam off. I came back up to the surface face up, and therefore didn't drown. I lay on top of the calm water in the bay and I thought this numbness in my body must go away. I felt detached from the lower part of my body, as if it were happening to somebody else. It was like when you've gone to sleep on your arm, then suddenly you wake up and your arm's completely numb, without power and sensation. I'd lost the rest of my body, and that was very weird. I'd knocked myself out as a kid diving into a settee at home; I'd got up and walked off, then fainted by the stairs. That had gone away, so I thought that this would too if I just lay there floating. But nothing happened, it didn't go away. I wasn't aware whether my hands worked or not at that time, but my arms moved, so I skulled on my back to the shore, lapping against the sandy beach like a log. I called to my friends whom I could vaguely see out of the corners of my eyes. I can't remember if I could move my head, but I could see something up the beach. They came down throwing sand at me, and although I was my usual flippant self, I said that I thought it was a bit more serious this time and they dragged me on to the beach. I was absolutely covered in sand. For some strange reason there was a doctor on the beach, who came and examined me, and sent off for the ambulance. I remember the doctor saying to me 'Are you all right?' and I said, 'Yes, except you're putting sand in my eyes,' – my usual self. They took me off to the local hospital, the old hospital, because the new one still wasn't built. I went to sleep there that night, and can't remember much about it. The next morning they told me that they couldn't find a radiologist, and were shipping me over to the main island on the ferry. To transfer me to the stretcher, they got five people round my bed and said, 'One, two, three, heave-ho' (but in their language), and the guy at my head lifted it first, so that probably did permanent extra damage. I felt pain then. We went across on the ferry in the ambulance to St Luke's Hospital on the main island of Malta. I stayed in the hospital there from 25th August, the day after the accident, and the day after my birthday, until 9th November. People, including a family friend who was a doctor, and my parents, said 'You must go to a specialist place called Stoke Mandeville.' I was lying there, waiting to get better and thought that a Maltese bed was as good as any other. Once the spinal shock had begun to wear off, I began to sense a bit more. Because my spinal cord was not completely damaged, some nerve messages began to get through. They didn't say, 'You know, this is it, mate, you're not going to walk again', so I assumed that things would change because they kept checking how much I could feel and whether there was any movement – there wasn't.

They stuck me in a little room on my own for which I had to pay (not an awful lot, because we had some sort of reciprocal arrangement). I had to pay extra for drugs and operations and all but the basics. Mr Amato, this lovely surgeon who'd actually been to Stoke Mandeville, as I learned later, was trying to protect me from paying too much money, because I wasn't insured, and there was no compensation in the pipeline. So he said things to me like 'Now we need to stretch the spinal column in the neck; the vertebrae normally sort themselves out and repair.' I can't remember exactly what he said, but he gave me options immediately, saying 'We can put you in halter traction or we can drill two holes in the side of your head, put a metal thing in and the weight on the cable going over the end of the bed can attach to that.' Being smart, and not having many brains anyway, I thought I'm not going to let them drill a couple of holes in the side of my head and let all my brains run out. So I chose what I thought was the right thing, the halter traction. Presumably he was happy that I accepted that, which meant he didn't have to give me an operation and charge me. So I started life as a disabled person making important decisions right away, but not realizing it. What happens to a lot of spinally injured people is that all decisions are taken away from them, but I started off making what were important decisions, even if the wrong ones, and for the wrong reasons. I didn't drink enough, developed mouth ulcers and became very thin because I wasn't eating enough. I didn't look at myself because I've never believed in looking at myself, so it didn't bother me but other people were a little worried. I was then flown out on 9 November by Casevac, the RAF evacuation service, which saved me some money. The occupational therapist happened to be a Brit, and her hubby was in the RAF, and she knew that the RAF have these planes which could fly you, so saving the cost of an ordinary flight.

I flew in a Hercules and we crept across Europe, just above the ground. We couldn't go over the Alps, we sort of went round them, so the views were absolutely wonderful. When we arrived at RAF Lyneham, it seemed to take days to land, as we descended through thick fog. We kept on going down and down and down, and I got this sensation, 'Bloody hell, we've missed the airport and we've missed the world!' Eventually we did land and I went by ambulance to Stoke Mandeville, not being able to afford to fly from RAF Lyneham by helicopter.

The next part could have been written by Kafka. There was me on this trolley that seemed to be roaring at a colossal speed down miles and miles of corridors with sudden flashes of different colours with white stripes on them – months later I discovered these were the fire doors. It just went on interminably, corridor after corridor, and then finally I arrived in a ward. Apparently they were really worried, expecting me to be in a really bad state as was often the case with people coming from overseas. There were pressure sores on my heels because they hadn't turned me from side to side in bed when I was in Malta, and I had bladder stones, but basically I was in remarkably good condition, presumably because I was an incomplete lesion.

A doctor examined me, but I sensed that to him I wasn't a human being. I felt like saying, 'Hey, this is me, I'm inside here!' They obviously thought I was in a very bad way, so they were checking me like you would check a faulty car: 'This moves' and 'This doesn't'... They were worried, and so they ignored the person and dealt with the immediately presenting problem which is obviously the way to do it. That night I felt desperately alone and lonely. The contrast with Malta was extreme: I'd been in a little room all on my own, and the physio used to come in to me at ten o'clock at night and tell me all her problems. She was a Scot, and I'd give her a cuddle, and we'd have a chat. She'd tell me all about the troubles she was having with her Maltese boyfriend, and she'd give me a bit of physio. A Maltese girl used to visit me every day, I don't know why – perhaps her mother told her it would be kind. She used to sit, and barely spoke, but would offer me a little something to eat. Friends had ensured that everybody who was crew on the Malta jet would pop in, so every few days some air hostess or steward used to call in and bring yet more Maltesers! Now I was lying in this ward in Stoke Mandeville and there was all this noise. I had just about got off to sleep, when suddenly there was pandemonium. I thought it must be morning, but it was dark. There were some lights down at the other end and voices roaring and shouting, then suddenly they came to my bed. I thought, 'What the hell's happening, this is a bloody madhouse!' They then came in talking and chatting, and moving me around, and giving an aperient, a laxative. I didn't know what it was and eventually went back to sleep again, but come fairly early morning when there was already some noise (they seemed to believe in noise in this place), suddenly I sensed that I was going to shit myself. Then, wham, I had. I never had anything like this over in Malta because they did it all the old-fashioned way, with soap and water and sticking a little pipe up my bum.

One of the things that a spinal unit does is to teach tetraplegics a tremendous amount about their body. In fact we know more about our body and how it operates than many GPs because, for instance, there are conditions like autonomic dysreflexia which are unique to us. Every so often at the Spinal Injuries Association, we hear of a GP who repeatedly makes a wrong diagnosis of a member, prescribes the wrong drugs or whatever for somebody who has autonomic dysreflexia, because they've never come across it before. That's one reason why we published our books, *So You're Paralysed* and *Treatment and Care for GPs and District Nurses*: in order to help our members know their own body so that they can help their GP understand their condition. They should also let their GP have the book as well, because often the GPs are not prepared to admit that the patients know more about their own condition than the GP does. It's vital that disabled people don't let GPs just over-rule them when they clearly don't understand the particular issue involved. Our spinal units do help us, and encourage us to understand our body, and we know that we can always ring up if we have problems.

Before the accident, I was working for a subsidiary of an American company. I had a flat up in Cumberland where we had a factory, and I used to travel around in the UK and Europe a bit, in technical sales. After my accident, they said I should come back. Before I'd had my accident I'd also started my own little business producing specialized printed circuits for cosmic ray chambers. I acted as a factor, getting other people to do the work, because the ordinary printed circuit manufacturers couldn't make big flexible circuits for cosmic-ray chambers. I carried on with that business while I was in hospital, just occasional orders which were farmed out. When I left hospital I decided not to return to Cumberland because I couldn't manage on my own. I was still learning to cope, and there were various things I couldn't manage on my own, so I went back to my parents' house in London. I'd always been interested in design so I developed contacts I knew in the trade and pursued print factoring, consultancy and typographical design. I used to enjoy working on artwork because, although my hands are gammy and I can't use scissors, I liked the challenge of trying to cut up bits of paper, sorting it all out and the satisfaction of eventually completing the artwork. I used to design catalogues and posters, for instance, for the Wildenstein Gallery in Bond Street, working with artists and translating their ideas into the appropriate style for their exhibition.

I'd do odd little jobs for charities and voluntary organizations, and knock something out for them. I did some book publishing, and published the Spinal Injuries Association's first book before joining the staff, *So You're Paralysed . . .* , in 1976. My fee was £100, and it cost me a fortune in time to launch that book, but I achieved great satisfaction from helping the Association. After publishing the book, when the Association's general secretary retired, I kept on going into the office because I was still promoting the book internationally. People kept on saying, 'You must take this job on, what's going to happen to SIA?' Eventually I applied for the job as organizing secretary and said, 'Well, I don't want this job actually, but if it's like this and this and this, I'll do it on a part-time basis because I've got my own company work'. After a lot more thinking they eventually decided to employ me as a development officer part-time.

I became the director of the SIA, and then executive director. We were one and a half people – I was the half person – and now the staff is just over thirty.

My survival motto has been, 'never take no for an answer'. Many people when they are told no, whether by a cinema manager or a benefits official, accept it. My attitude was that you do what you want and have to do. When I was in Stoke Mandeville I wasn't one of those good patients, I wasn't somebody who sat there quietly when I was given the wrong pill.

I think it is very important that disabled people learn from each other, not just those with spinal cord injury. You meet people who have been to a special school where they've been denied social interaction with their peers and conditioned to low expectations; you meet them as young disabled people when they wouldn't say boo to a goose; and then you meet them five years later and they could chew you up and spit you out in little pieces!

You also need a particularly good set of social skills when you are disabled. The average able-bodied person has very bad social skills and, because of this, you as a disabled person need to develop extremely good social skills in order to operate effectively in a world designed for able-bodied people and help them to behave normally. They get in such a mess, trying to work out what to do when they meet disabled people: they don't know whether to sit on the floor or crouch, or at what angle to crane their necks. It's wonderful meeting able-bodied people who are just totally natural and naturally get to the same level as you. I already had those sorts of basic social skills because of my background. However, many disabled people, because they don't grow alongside their able-bodied peers, don't develop good social skills until they get out of special schools. It's the same with able-bodied people with bad social skills: if they have a spinal-cord injury, it takes them a while to get to grips, not just with their physical impairment, but to realize that it's the able-bodied people who have the problem and don't know how to behave. Because able-bodied people are the norm, the majority, they don't realize they have a problem and that they create the hostile attitudinal and environmental barriers which actually make disabled people's lives more difficult. In some ways, as I see it, it's the same with women and men: women have been put down so much by men that they accept the blame for all the problems, "everything's the woman's fault". I think disabled people have basically got it right, and have to help these poor able-bodied people to sort themselves out.

Since the early Seventies I have attended various disability seminars and conferences and given talks. I was my usual outspoken self and used to be brought in to address bureaucratic nonsense and those crazy things that we have had to put up with over the years. The general public are only now beginning to understand what it's all about. The debate on the Civil Rights Disabled Persons Bill in the House of Commons on 11 March 1994 was much more sophisticated than the first debate on anti-discrimination legislation back in 1984. The understanding of our position in society has moved on, and this is very much because disabled people have identified for themselves what their situation is rather than accepting the traditional view which has been imposed on them. We have rejected the individual or medical model of disability in favour of the social model. Disability is no longer seen as a problem caused by our impairment, but a relationship between the individual and an often hostile environment, which may prevent us living an ordinary everyday life. Society to me has been created by men aged between twenty and thirty, fit and healthy people who can leap on to a bus and never push a pram. The majority of the population, however, aren't into formulating our society and creating our environment, and that's why kitchens, houses and so on were designed for men, not for women or children or old people. This runs through the whole of the environment; it's structured for fit young men. If we team up with women and old people, we are the majority, and then we might see an environment created for everybody, one where disabled people are not excluded, from integrated education to employment opportunities.

In a spinal unit you're caught between the individual plus personal tragedy model and the social model of disability. While you emerge from the individual model of disability where they're trying to modify you, working on you to make you fit into the environment, they are also trying to equip you with skills so that you can manage on your own as a wheelchair user, for which you need the right wheelchair, an accessible house and an income, etc. I wasn't able to articulate that in a structured way in some of my early articles and talks.

I'd been to the States in 1974, after the Rehabilitation Act had come through there, in 1973. I'd talked to this black tetraplegic guy about the black experience, and I began to see that we'd have to change our approach from condescension to rights. But how was this possible in a country that had no constitution embodying rights, a country where the concept of rights was alien? It wasn't until people like Paul Hunt and Vic Finkelstein began to revolutionize the thinking on disability, and then Mike Oliver created a framework, that I realized my ideas were floating around there, but 'lost', if you like. Vic used one of the articles I wrote in 1978 for the *Nursing Times* as a sort of think-piece for an early Open University course: he told me about all these bright students, much brighter than me, who didn't know what I was talking and writing about because the concepts were so new to them. In that article I talked of the need for rights legislation.

The thing that I very much recognize is how lucky I am. You meet other people whose spouse has caused the accident, or for whom this went wrong or that went wrong, or whose family cried every time they met them – you hear really dreadful stories. Whereas, even though mine was a terrible experience, it wasn't that terrible for me. It was probably a lot worse for my parents, although they appeared to manage it extremely well.

Even on Malta, it wasn't this huge problem as I had friends around who stayed on a bit longer after our holiday, and my parents came over. The accident was also entirely my own fault, so I didn't have to blame anybody. At Stoke Mandeville I had a smashing physio, and I met people who took me out of the unit on visits and pub crawls. It wasn't as awful as for some people who had medical complications or family problems. Neither was I racked with pain. I did have to have an op after I came back from Malta to remove bladder stones.

There was a period when I was always covered in sweat after getting dressed in the morning. This was caused by my bladder not emptying that brilliantly. Eventually they gave me another op, a resection of the bladder neck to make the pee flow a bit better, after which I wasn't soaking wet from sweat any more. Now I don't sweat at all unless my bladder's too full; it's all to do with my autonomic nervous system, and nothing to do with being too hot.

I also was lucky getting into sport. Before my accident I had enjoyed and played tennis and hockey regularly, but not to a high standard. Now, in a wheelchair, I found I was quite good at table tennis. When I left hospital I began to play regularly at the Stoke Mandeville Paraplegic Athletics Club. My ability to manage alone as a tetraplegic developed by watching the other guys – we all slept in a hut – and checking how they did things, asking them how to cope when staying with other people, and so on. In fact when I was still in hospital I wanted to stay with this girl, and I said, 'Look, I can't go with this great big Winchester bottle and all these pipes and things, this is ridiculous'. I asked this guy from the great outside who I'd met playing table tennis and he said, 'Oh, no, you don't want to worry about all that. What you do is this, this, this and this.' So I learned from spinally injured people the art of actually living outside because they were living with it. You only got so much information fed back through the system, so when I left the spinal unit I said that what was needed was a manual full of practical advice. That's something that I've been waiting over twenty years to do and the SIA has now produced what I needed then.

Shortly after I left, I entered the Stoke Mandeville national games and came second in the table tennis, plus I didn't do too badly in the archery. They said, 'Right, you're off to the Olympics.' I was thinking that this cripple lark isn't too bad really, is it? When you come out, it's all so awful and desperate, yet things weren't that bad for me after all. My business was bringing in a bit of money. I had no accident compensation payment pending, but I was doing these sports, and here they are saying, 'Right, off to Israel.' So I went to the Paralympics and won a bronze for archery and after that I went into the games in most years up until about 1980. I took a silver medal for archery and a couple of bronzes in 1972 in

Heidelberg for table tennis, and then in 1976 in Toronto I won the gold for table tennis and the team gold with my mate, who was brilliant. I also went to New Zealand for the Commonwealth Games in 1974.

I was earning a living and travelling the world, and thus being a wheelchair user was a very positive experience in many ways for me. It wasn't as bad as it is or can be for very many people. I also had lucky breaks which other people didn't have.

Obviously I've had lots of failures, but they are all relative. Basically, at the time I came out of hospital I was already getting on with things and there were enough positive experiences to counter the negative ones. You might stop and think, 'Hey, it would be nice to kick the leaves in autumn, wouldn't it?', but you don't say, 'Oh God, if only I could kick the leaves in autumn.' Becoming depressed is something that you can easily fall into, I think, depending on the sort of person you are, and on the circumstances. I didn't have a colossal negative picture building up, and therefore it was easier for me to get on with things.

For instance, sex was something I enjoyed and because I can feel over the surface of my body, sex is still great fun to me. OK, there are still problems with it: you have to empty your bladder, so you can't be spontaneous. In some ways I was more squeamish and hung up about sex than some of the other guys I was in hospital with, often more severely disabled, but nothing stopped them. You think, 'well, what the hell am I hanging about for?' That's one of the great advantages of a spinal unit: it's always forgotten that actually what it is all about is learning to live out there in the big wide world, and you learn most from your peer group. So when Fred or whoever, who was more severely disabled than you, just got on and did things, you thought, 'If he can do all those sorts of things, I must stop being such a weed.'

It's up to disabled people themselves to take charge of the situation and share their bright outlook on life with the able-bodied people. That's what's so important about social skills, because if disabled people can master the situation, it's fascinating how quickly the wheelchair becomes irrelevant. You see so many of our members, women and men with their children, and it's just wonderful and beautiful, so easy and relaxed. There weren't any hang-ups, they just got on with it.

Funnily enough, when I was about seventeen, I was at a co-educational school. A group of us always used to be debating things, and I said I didn't want children for all sorts of reasons, and wasn't worried whether I got married or not. I have been unofficially engaged to a physiotherapist, and since I've been in a wheelchair, quite a number of people have wanted to marry me, but I still don't want to get married. There's this idea that, because you are in a wheelchair, you're rejected by all the able-bodied people or it's only the kinky people that are after you, which is nonsense. When I was in New Zealand, in Dunedin for the Paraplegic Games, I met this really interesting woman. Chatting to her in the pub, I didn't realize how tall she was. I suddenly realized why she was travelling round the world on her own: although a very attractive Canadian blonde, she was about six foot three tall, and so she didn't 'fit' in many ways. I suppose she found it easy to identify with us.

That question of size is actually quite fascinating because, after being in a wheelchair for a relatively short time in Stoke Mandeville, all the physiotherapists were tall people, *everybody* was taller. It was so funny when I stood up on callipers for the first time and suddenly realized that this strong and wonderful physiotherapist who had lifted me up, thrown me around, pushed me in the water, and slung me over her shoulder, only came up to my nipples. To me it's fascinating how slowly human beings change their gut attitudes, yet at the same time how rapidly we perceive change in others and how quickly we can adopt an entirely new perspective of something after relatively short exposure.

Coping with the 'practicalities' of life – such as bowel function – can be one of the most humiliating experiences if you let it get to you. When I was a novice disabled person, I had a couple of ghastly accidents with my bowels, and in front of other people. At the time it's absolutely terrible and impossible and you feel you cannot live a second more, because of the total humiliation. But then you put it aside and start the next day with a smile. That's what you've got to do. Life doesn't end when something goes wrong. However bad it looks in your mind, life goes on, so you've got to stamp on it, learn from it, put it aside and try again. That's why working is often so important to so many disabled people: you've got to do things, you've got to go for it the whole time just like anybody else. The difference between able-bodied and disabled is often exaggerated – it's as if we are a different race or something – but when you analyse all the experiences, they are actually very similar in terms of how human beings react and what they do about it. I always remember a friend of mine, a sculptor who used to earn a living doing building works, rushing into my house one day, and he sort of shat himself. So even able-bodied people have problems like that. We are not a different race, and these are general human experiences: because people happen to be in wheelchairs or happen to be blind or deaf doesn't suddenly make them aliens.

Tremendous advances have been made in the understanding of how the spinal cord tries to re-grow. Obviously a lot has been learned about the spinal cord, and this may be of particular use immediately after an accident. For instance methyl prednisalone is now used regularly after spinal cord injury because all the evidence is that it reduces the severity of the permanent injury to the nerves. This new understanding increases our ability to reduce the severity of the spinal cord injury damage. There is some evidence to suggest that, by the year 2000, we will be able to achieve functional laboratory rejoining of nerves. It's been done in Japan for instance, on newborn rats, but a newborn rat is very different to a human being with a mature established spinal cord which no longer readily regenerates. There are all manner of complications and toxins which tend to inhibit re-growth, which must be understood and mastered before experiments can start on humans.

Although welcoming the benefits of research, I don't live with false expectations of what might come in a few years' time, and that I'll be up and running about, because it isn't like that. It may entail operations, and I might die from the anaesthetic. OK, I have the operation and it's successful, and I get a bit of movement back in my legs. I then undergo rehabilitation for a long time. But what if I'm racked with pain after some nerves rejoin? It's not for me, but newly-injured people in the next century may well benefit. Talk of 'curing' disabled people all too easily reinforces negative stereotypes of us as worthless or lesser beings, unemployable or a drain on society, rather than fostering positive images of us as real people, contributing, full citizens who pay their taxes. It helps the public think that we are better people if we stand up, or that if we stand up we are 'cured'. If you can function better on callipers than in a wheelchair, great, but I think there's no point in just standing up for the sake of it, or acceding to this idea that you are a better man if you are standing. I can stand up on callipers, but I can't take a step or do anything else at the same time.

For me, research into managing pain is of prime importance. I don't experience much pain myself but I talk to people with intractable pain and hear what they go through. Pain is 100 times worse than the fact that you can't walk, and if you said I could walk with the same pain or be in a wheelchair with no pain, I know which I'd choose, give me freedom from severe pain every time. Pain is a problem that I'm trying to address at the Spinal Injuries Association here and now with a major research programme. Whatever happens in the future, pain is the single most debilitating side effect of paraplegia. For those with bad pain, it's absolutely devastating, and that is why alleviating pain is my particular research crusade.

Able-bodied people tend to assume that the overriding wish of all those with spinal injuries is to be able to walk again. There is a major problem in the imposing of able-bodied norms on disabled people. The fact that I can't walk actually isn't the problem, it is the inaccessible environment and people's attitudes. People can manage perfectly well in a wheelchair, but it's all the other things that are the problem: pain, or the fact that able-bodied people say, 'I saw so and so standing up. When are you going to be standing up and walking?' or 'Have you lost faith and hope about ever walking again?' Able-bodied people impose such views on disabled people, rather than accepting disabled people's experience and perspective on living with an impairment. Different disabled people make different judgements about what is right or wrong for them, and what their hopes and expectations are in life. Some people's reason for living is to await the day when they are up and walking, while others say, 'I don't believe I'll ever walk again'. Members of the Spinal Injuries Association hold a total spectrum of views, but we don't want other people imposing on disabled people their culture and views, because disabled people are developing their own understanding of their situation, their own perspective of what's happened to them. They've come to view the world differently from able-bodied people, and all this concentration on trying to 'modify' them so they can do this and that is all very well but actually the problem is the hostile physical and attitudinal environment in which we live.

If we were to talk in ideal terms about what would be good for disabled people, I would say you've got to revise the whole ablist culture that is around us, from the way the Bible portrays disabled people, all the way through to PR and advertising, which portrays an anti-physical impairment approach. You're either a superhero, courageously overcoming adversity, or pathetic, or tragic. Then again, if you're visually impaired you can get more money begging. In some countries, people actually disable their kids so that they can earn more money. In this reverse logic it actually is positive to be disabled because you can get better income than an able-bodied person in that society. There are all sorts of confused images, but within our society the basic thing is the negative stereotypes that are pumped out the whole time, not just at disabled people, it's the body beautiful thing. These images oppress most people within society because we all fall short of ideal. But for disabled people there's not just the body beautiful, there's all the other negative imagery that is piled on.

Because disabled people fall short of the ideal in a number of respects they are pigeonholed: the human mind has this way of labelling someone and once you've labelled them and they're in the pigeonhole, it's incredibly difficult for them to escape and be the ordinary, everyday human beings they are in reality. Disability is a human rights issue, not a medical problem, so we should help people escape out of these pigeonholes, and admit we're all in it together. It's the negative imagery which devalues the status of being a disabled person, so one needs to counter that in the same way that you say black is beautiful. But it is very difficult to persuade people when the sale of the product is the be all and end all of advertising. Yet what is fascinating is how quickly you can turn the negative imagery around if there is the will. In the States, the McDonalds chain has ads with a family with a wheelchair user, an ad for the whole of the community, and suddenly disability and a family with a wheelchair user become ordinary, everyday and acceptable. Immediately, we're just ordinary people living ordinary lives. The media has great difficulty in selling ordinary people, so TV and radio programmes present us as either pathetic or super heroic, you've either got to be really ugly or really beautiful. The piles of myths perpetuated in literature, and in the Bible, are all part of our culture, and some are based on genuine facts of life. But how do you stop them being seen as negative and get them accepted as just an ordinary part of life, so that disabled people don't have to get up every single day and counter these negative stereotypes. That's why disability is a struggle for many people because they're having to fight issues the whole time, they're having to gain entry to cinemas, they're having to fight with the manager, and nobody's on their side. This is why, early on, I used to argue about access and fire regulations: the onus shouldn't be on me to persuade the manager to admit me.

I worked on a booklet with the National Consumer Council called *Getting Around: The Beginner's Guide to Access for Disabled People 1981*. This covered the whole question of access to public places like cinemas and theatres. Fire regulations were always used as an excuse to keep us out, yet there hadn't been a fatal accident in a cinema for twenty-five years. My quote summed up the great fire hazard: 'Anyone would think we spontaneously ignite!' Not until we have comprehensive legislation to outlaw unjustifiable discrimination will the need to fight for the simple right to enter a cinema disappear.

As for the benefit system, I'm a member and chairman of my local group of the Disablement Income Group. Way back in the late Sixties, DIG highlighted the fact that there were no benefits at all for married women, and fought for and achieved provision, and it was also DIG that won the attendance allowance. It was they that began the huge strides forward that enabled severely disabled people to escape from institutions into the community because for the first time, they controlled money. We still need an effective national disability income covering the extra expenses of disability tax free and a taxable pension element. The system isn't really helpful in getting disabled people back to work because the pension element does not taper off gradually as your earnings increase. There's a huge jump from unemployed to employed. The system still doesn't provide adequate benefits for very severely disabled people. It's very important that the Spinal Injuries Association takes particular care to protect the interests of its most severely disabled members, those with the biggest physical impairments, because the have the greatest expenses. Every time there's a review, the tendency is to spread the butter a bit more thinly – statistically, it looks better to help more people. This tendency must be resisted, otherwise very severely disabled people will be forced back into institutions. We have to protect selected groups within the disability movement, otherwise they will simply be excluded and their rights to a full life denied.

I'm chairman of Rights Now!, the group of voluntary organizations for anti-discrimination legislation. Way back in 1978 I wrote an article calling for rights legislation when 'rights' was a dirty word, and it's only now, at last, that talk of rights is accepted and for the first time the word was used in a parliamentary Bill (the Civil Rights (Disabled Persons) Bill). This is the single most important piece of legislation this century and would give disabled people the right to do everyday things. People will no longer be able to say 'You can't do this' and 'You can't do that', and to do so without giving a reason. It would be the beginning of the end of unjustifiable discrimination against disabled people.

We are making some progress. I've been fighting for access to the London Underground for years. I was a member of the London Regional Passengers' Committee and before that the TUCC for London. Now they have accepted that the decision whether or not to use the Underground is up to the disabled person. London Underground will give me a map of the accessible and inaccessible stations, and then it's my judgement as to whether I go or not. There'll be no guards running after me and saying 'Oh sorry, you're not allowed on'. I'm now in control, and this is a remarkable change. It's that sort of new thinking which will revolutionize our experience as disabled people.

Gaining access is a continuous fight for each disabled person, a fight which we should not have to endure. You win one fight against the fire regulations, then the next hurdle is insurance. You win accessible taxis, but what of accessible public places? Then you achieve secondary legislation changes, then you change primary legislation . . . . Whereas if you have rights legislation, there is a fundamental change which will enable disabled people to do things unfettered by phoney excuses, and to have the sense of their right to do them. To me it will also demolish that feeling of alienation which disabled people have, that they are excluded from so much of society. Every day they have to struggle against the odds and the enactment of the civil rights Bill would make a lot of disabled people feel, 'I've got a right to be here, I've become a citizen of this country, I actually now have a right to exist.' This legislation would not just mean accessible public transport, for example, it would change the thinking of disabled people about themselves and their right to be equal and full citizens of this country. Of course it would also change the attitudes of all these poor able-bodied people who don't realize that they are the problem because they are the majority. Once disabled people are out there in the community, travelling on the bus to work with all these able-bodied people, public attitudes to us will change, as has happened in other countries which already have anti-discrimination legislation.

I want integrated education, not just so that disabled people can integrate and react with their peer group, but because I believe that disabled people could have a good influence on these violent kids and perhaps might help to develop a less violent society. If we were properly integrated, you could perhaps develop a much more understanding community. Instead of pigeonholing disabled people, looking at us as a special group who need separate, special schools, special housing, special transport, special employment; we should be seen as, and become, part of a whole integrated society.

Disabled people do not just experience direct discrimination that you can see quite straightforwardly – you can't get on a bus or into a pub –

but institutionalized discrimination which is caused by the very way our society is structured. I've talked about special schools already: where the regime conditions people to have low expectations, you discriminate unjustifiably against them by making them less able to compete for work and so on. They start off discriminated against, and then they can't use public transport, therefore you provide them with special segregated buses; you then employ them in sheltered workshops because they haven't the opportunity to gain open employment or develop good social skills. Then perhaps at the age of thirty they emerge from all this enforced conditioning realizing that they're intelligent people, may go and get further qualifications and become more integrated people. But they've lost ten years of their life because society has structured itself to prevent them getting a proper education and growing up like any other kid on the block. They had been siphoned off and put in pigeonholes.

When you look at discrimination against black people, particularly in the States, and how they rose up to confront the issue, it's the same type of cause and effect as we are experiencing, and we are learning from them how to overcome the problem. What Martin Luther King did in the States for black people, followed by the demonstrations and so forth, enabled disabled people in the United States to unite and fight. Other minority groups joined their campaign and now they have comprehensive anti-discrimination legislation in the form of the Americans with Disabilities Act passed in 1990.

For a long time after I first worked for SIA, I didn't take real holidays, because there was just too much to do. I used to take a couple of weeks off to compete in the National Games. I was lucky enough to travel abroad for the Olympic Games, although I was still talking about disability and persuading people to join the SIA. Now I take my holidays, and I tend to try and go somewhere warm in March, like Lanzarote or Cyprus. I don't go on holiday in the summer, because it's usually so beautiful and wonderful here in the UK, but at the end of October or beginning of November, I might go somewhere warmer again.

I live on my own now, although the flat upstairs is where my mother and brother live, and I do do some housework myself. I occasionally get somebody in to do a complete 'spring clean', but my method is that if I don't make too much mess, I don't have too much to clear up. I occasionally attempt the vacuuming and quite enjoy a bit of cooking. Sorting out the plants, with my tetraplegic hands, is a bit of a challenge, and I'll spend hours at the weekend repotting – only occasionally, mind you.

I drive my own car, and am able to pull my wheelchair into it on my own, which is great. I occasionally take trains and I find them absolutely excellent: they're fast and usually cheaper than going by car. I loved travelling by bus when I was in Vancouver, just because they are accessible and you're on public transport like anyone else, but I haven't tried any of the new scheduled accessible bus services in our country. I have used Dial-A-Ride, and I tried the Airbus to and from Heathrow Airport just to see how it works. I've used taxis over the years; the new ones are certainly much easier, because you enter in your wheelchair rather than via the floor with a heave and a shove. I take the view that if I need to be somewhere, nothing will stop me. I think it's very important for people to accept that some experiences are frustrating, difficult, embarrassing or whatever, but that you have to put this aside as something you've just got to go through. Your target, after all, is not the bus ride or the taxi ride, it's actually to meet a client, or get to the pub to meet your friends.

I used to exercise by planned pushes around the block or in the park, but these days my excuse is lack of time, or is it age? Nowadays, I'm exhausted pushing from the office to my car, and from my car into my home! When I'm on holiday, I might suddenly say, 'Right, I'm going to take some exercise', and push three times round the swimming pool, or actually take a swim.

To anyone in a similar position to mine I'd say: Never take no for an answer. Get up and go, do what you want. OK, listen to other people, and learn from what they say, but ultimately it's your decision as to how you run your life. You must make sure that you control your own life, decide for yourself what risks to take, and do what you want to do: there is no-one else who can live your life for you. Your life is up to you and you can achieve what others think is impossible. The world is your oyster.

Useful Addresses

Spinal Injuries Association
Newpoint House
76 St James's Lane
London N10 3DF
Tel: (0181) 441 2121

The Spinal Injuries Association is the national organization for spinal cord injured people and their families. Run by paralyzed people, the SIA offers through first-hand experience a wealth of practical information and advice about living with spinal cord injury. For further information please contact the above address.

International Spinal Research Trust
100 Crossbrook Street
Cheshunt
Herts EN8 8JJ
Tel: (01992) 641999